WALL PILATES WORKOUTS

FOR WOMEN OVER 50

Your Gentle 4-Week Program of Home Workouts for Balance, Back Pain Relief, Joint Health, Flexibility, and Core Strength With Over 50+ Illustrated Exercises

LAUREN BIRCH

Contents

Introduction

Aging can feel like a difficult path, and aging as a woman comes with a number of issues. As we approach our 50s, health considerations turn from healthy weight and fertility to changing hormones, ailing strength, and muscle and bone degeneration.

Our nutritional needs begin to change, we ache in places we didn't know existed, and don't get me started on what happens with a simple cough, sneeze, or giggle, let alone try to deadlift 50 pounds in the gym! Our bodies seem to tell us that we're slowing down, that now is the time to set aside the heavy weight and embrace a new strength-building dawn, but not many of us know how to transition into this new era of health and fitness.

This is where Wall Pilates comes in. It's a gateway to enhanced well-being for women, like you who are looking for thoughtful exercise practices that are specifically designed for our newly evolving bodies.

Wall Pilates is more than mere movement and strength building, it's a synergy of graceful motion, intentional breathing, and mindfulness that centers on utilizing the wall for support and resistance. Each movement learned and practiced brings us closer to becoming attuned to our changing bodies, and empowers us to renew our strength, reclaim our bodies, and lay the foundation for independence as we move into our golden years.

What makes Wall Pilates different from conventional workouts is the way in which it hones balance and poise. By working stabilizer muscles, and adapting our workouts to suit specific limitations, we can work with our bodies so that we're no longer pushing through persistent aches, pains, and questionable balance. Instead, Wall Pilates provides us with manageable, effective workouts that fit within our routines without demanding a drastic reshuffling of our existing schedule and health and fitness goals.

Before we dive into what you can expect from *Wall Pilates for Women Over 50*, I'd like to share a story about Sarah, a friend of mine who has been in my life throughout, what seems like, every phase. From high school romances, and breakups, to marriage, kids, and careers, Sarah has been an ever-present guiding light in my life. So, as we approached 50, and I seemed to miss out on most of the nasty transitional changes of life, it pained me to see one of my best friends suffer through pain and discomfort.

Sarah had always juggled multiple roles, wife, mother, homebody, and corporate extraordinaire but as 50 approached and went, she felt the unmistakable signs of aging creeping in. Her once-familiar agility was giving way to subtle stiffness, and persistent back pain that hindered a lot of things she could once do with ease. To add insult to injury, hot flushes and a growing pillow of fat, despite her best efforts to eat well, hindered her attempts at staying fit and healthy even further.

But, Sarah has never been one to submit to any onslaught and together, we found the solution—Wall Pilates! With renewed hope, we set about creating a four-week workout plan, ways to track our progress, and tweaked our nutrition to nourish our bodies. Somewhere around week three, Sarah bent down to pick up a dog toy and as she stood upright, she smiled. "I haven't been able to do that without pain in years!" The results were clear! Wall Pilates, persistence, and nutrition worked.

Sarah's journey to a healthy, well-nourished, and pain-free body needed to be shared—as did my weight loss and newly svelte body, and that is why I chose to write this book.

Over the upcoming chapters, you can expect to learn

- the basics of wall Pilates, including warm-up and cool-down stretches to keep your body supple and injury-free.

- focused exercise routines that allow you to work on the aspects of your fitness, flexibility, and balance that matter most to you.

- advancing wall Pilates programs that take you from beginner to advanced at your own pace.

- safe deep stretches and wall Pilates moves that help strengthen your core, alleviate back pain, and work stabilizer muscles for better balance and posture.

- advice on changing nutritional needs including how to eat for your hormones and your wellness.

- and so much more.

Wall Pilates is so much more than a home workout, it's an accessible way to achieve your personal fitness goals, build resilience, and live a balanced life that embraces well-being as we age.

With over illustrations to help you perfect your movements, breathing guidance for mindful engagement, and tips and tricks for mental well-being and pain management, *Wall Pilates for Women Over 50* is your comprehensive guide to a healthy, pain-free transition into your golden years.

The Pillars of Wall Pilates for Women Over 50

The first step to a stronger, more flexible self is to first know what you're aiming to achieve with Wall Pilates, and then to know what Wall Pilates can do for you. For those entering their sixties or already navigating this empowering decade, it's vital to focus on exercises that strengthen the body but also to not neglect our mental and emotional well-being. The foundational aspects of Wall Pilates align with these concepts because it encourages precision and mindfulness over intensity and the brute force of our past workouts.

Instead, Wall Pilates focuses on fluidity, breath, and mental engagement as the foundation for gains in strength, mobility, and flexibility. Added to this, Wall Pilates is accessible to everyone who has a wall, a sturdy chair, and the chutzpah to invest some time into their health and well-being.

Chapter 1 focuses on what Wall Pilates is and how it can benefit your health and well-being. It takes you on a journey into the history of Pilates, explains the fundamentals of the exercise, and highlights the benefits to you.

While you may not be actively doing any exercise in this chapter, you will be preparing yourself both physically and mentally for engaging in a safe and productive Wall Pilates routine. Now, before you begin with any exercise, I'd like you to remember that your safety and security are crucial. Make sure that you're consulting with a healthcare practitioner if you have limitations or if you have led a sedentary couple of years.

Understanding Wall Pilates

Pilates as a practice was developed and pioneered by Joseph Pilates. The Pilates method was first conceived in the early 20th century with the intent of achieving muscle control through mental focus, centering on the powerhouses of core strength and flexibility.

Growing up, Joseph was a sickly child. He suffered from rickets and chronic asthma and his small, sickly stature made him an easy target for bullies. One encounter with a bully left him blind in his left eye, but despite the adversities he faced, Joseph was determined to find a way to become healthy.

By age 12, Joseph became fascinated with human anatomy, exploring the physical form and seeking to understand how flow and breath exercises like yoga and martial arts produced more strength and muscle-defining results than other, more rigorous workouts.

By 14, Joseph delved into the world of Eastern wellness practices and began to understand the power of breath and mindfulness when it came to developing muscle strength. With this new understanding, he set about developing a new system of exercise—one that was accessible to people with physical limitations as well as healthy individuals. While early forms of the exercise weren't necessarily well-received, a few short years later, Pilates took the world of rehabilitation by storm.

Today, Pilates has been adapted to take on many shapes and forms, with Wall Pilates being a distinct variation specifically engineered to underpin the shifting physical requirements of older adults.

Central to Wall Pilates is the use of a simple wall as a constant and reliable environmental element. The wall is used as your primary support apparatus when completing your exercises and allows you to perform movements with confidence. Added to this, the addition of a wall to traditional Pilates movements minimizes the stress placed on your joints and takes pressure off the lower and mid-back.

While some equipment can be used to elevate your Wall Pilates workouts, elaborate equipment simply isn't necessary. Light-weight dumbbells can be replaced with water bottles, and otherwise expensive yoga mats can be substituted with already-owned non-slip shower mats. This makes Wall Pilates truly one of the most accessible exercises for people from all walks of life.

What Wall Pilates does *not* do is deviate from the central powerful focus of the Pilates discipline—breath and controlled movement. The introduction of a wall to your Pilates workout does, however, offer more tactile resistance, contributes toward correct body alignment, and enables you to internalize the crucial Pilates principles of centrality, focus, control, precision, and breathing.

Wall Pilates safely integrates the fundamental principles of Pilates, allowing you to progress as your core and stabilizer muscles strengthen. This means you can progress in strength much quicker than more traditional weight-lifting exercises, increasing your resistance easily while you grow stronger.

What you need to remember with any form of Pilates is that precision and moderation when carrying out movements are absolutely key to injury prevention and adequate strength, balance, and flexibility gains. Wall Pilates is a deliberate act that reinforces the core's engagement and activates the tiny muscle groups needed for balance and overall mobility.

The Benefits of Wall Pilates For Women Over 50

Crossing into the years beyond sixty brings with it a sharpened focus on selecting fitness routines that bolster our vitality. Wall Pilates offers a host of meaningful benefits that can enrich our lives as we mature and undergo a new set of changes to our bodies.

Before we dive into the benefits of Wall Pilates, I'd like to commend you on your commitment to reclaiming your body and health. Deciding to begin a Wall Pilates daily exercise routine goes beyond a mere commitment to staying fit. It introduces you to the concept that growing older doesn't mean having to slow down and give up the things you enjoy. In fact, Wall Pilates may encourage you to recapture some of those youthful practices you enjoyed being shelved in favor of your career, kids, or other life responsibilities!

Bone Health

Wall Pilates improves muscle tone and using the wall as a stabilizer adds a considerable amount of resistance to your workout. This added resistance engages muscles more strategically and the hallmark deliberate movements ensure the body begins to strengthen in a balanced and more synchronized manner than traditional exercise.

An emphasis on weight-bearing exercises promotes the reinforcement of bone density, acting as a countermeasure against osteoporosis, an issue many women over 50 face. Additionally, Wall Pilates encourages proprioception—an awareness of body position and movement—fortifying balance and reducing the likelihood of falls.

Emotional Well-Being

The emotional well-being of women post-fifty often becomes complex. Plummeting hormones and a different set of responsibilities and duties can bring with it stress and managing anxiety becomes of utmost importance.

Wall Pilates becomes a tranquil refuge that guides you through breathing and mindfulness techniques that extend beyond the benefits of traditional exercises. The mindful movements curate a meditative quietness that helps ease tension and promote serenity. I've lost count of how many women have told me that the transformative nature of Wall Pilates in their lives centered more around stress management than anything else.

Of course, a confidence boost from a stronger, leaner, and more supple body doesn't hurt, but it's the inherent mindful movement of Wall Pilates that packs a powerful mental health punch.

Resilience and Adaptability

There is a good reason that doctors, rehab specialists, and caretakers endorse the use of Wall Pilates as a go-to exercise after the age of 50. The exercise is adaptable and provides a sustainable, manageable way for people with mobility limitations a chance to build strength, manage pain, and be in total control of the movement of their body.

Wall Pilates builds resilience, keeps you thinking on your toes, and allows you to adapt your workouts to suit your needs. The less demanding nature of Wall Pilates means recovery times are greatly reduced and more active time is spent working out.

Hormonal Balance

Let me preface this chapter by saying exercise alone will not regulate hormonal changes but it can help! Everything from stress reduction to improved sleep helps to regulate cortisol levels in the body, reducing the negative effects of the stress and anxiety accompanied by the "change of life." Because chronic stress can contribute to hormonal imbalances, by managing stress, Pilates may indirectly support hormonal balance.

The reduction in fat, specifically belly fat can help to further manage hormonal imbalances, and improve heart health and circulation in the process. Decreasing estrogen can lead to symptoms of brain fog that are greatly improved by dopamine, serotonin, and stored estrogen being released into the bloodstream. All of this enhances mood, calming those sometimes dramatic mood swings we become prone to as we transition out of menopause and enter into a post-menopausal state.

Safety Guidelines & Injury Prevention

When taking on any fitness routine, especially once we get a bit older, it's important that we take our safety into account. While the information in this section is not meant to replace a professional healthcare provider's advice, it will serve as an introduction to the crucial safety protocols required to safely practice Wall Pilates. Some of this advice is practical and other of it will need to be used with discernment as you assess your own limitations.

It's important to acknowledge and respect your body's present capabilities and of course, with maturity comes a nuanced awareness of your body. Having said that, there may be times when you forget that 50 has come and gone, and you may be tempted to ramp things up before you're ready. The beauty of Wall Pilates is that it offers the flexibility to customize your practice. Don't overdo things, progress at your comfort level and within a range of motion that feels right for you.

Right, with that out of the way, let's get into the nitty-gritty of how to be safe while practicing Wall Pilates.

During your exercise routine, you'll be using a wall as a versatile assistive tool for balance, stability, and resistance. You're going to need to select a wall area that is devoid of any hindrances or hangings. This provides you with a safe and reliable surface against which you can execute your exercises.

Take into consideration the texture of the wall—smoother surfaces may seem beneficial but may lack grip for some movements. Conversely, movements that require you to slide might require a more smooth surface.

As you interact with the wall during your exercises you may feel a little strange. This is because the wall educates you about your body's alignment, indicating the correct positioning of the spine, shoulders, and weight distribution. The feedback from the wall is invaluable in ascertaining whether or not you're executing a move correctly.

The guiding rule for Wall Pilates is pain-free movement. If it feels painful or if you're unbalanced, readjust until you're more comfortable. Wall Pilates is designed to contribute positively to your health, not to challenge it unduly, or make you feel like you're doing something wrong. Take pauses, be mindful of your form, and adapt where necessary.

Finally, while I've done my best to offer modifications to exercises, feel free to tailor the Wall Pilates exercises provided. If your legs are particularly strong but your core needs some work, mix and match to customize your approach to fitness.

Above all else, be gentle with yourself and employ a little humor in your workouts. Wall Pilates isn't meant to be a drag—it's a celebration of your current capabilities and the anticipation of what you will be capable of. Approach your workouts with curiosity, put some music on, and pay attention to what you're doing; and you'll be stronger and fitter than you thought you could be sooner than you think.

Setting Up Your Workout Space

Once you've chosen a suitable wall, you can set up your space. To remain safe, and ensure you don't have to stop and start your workouts, having a clutter-free, well-organized space is important.

Begin by clearing your space of any clutter and furniture you may bump into. Some people choose to have a dedicated workout space but any wall that doesn't contain a radiator and has easily removable furniture is perfectly fine. Corner spaces are particularly handy for beginners to Wall Pilates as the adjacent solid surface minimizes the risk of falling.

Next, gather any equipment you feel you might need. This could be resistance bands if you're looking for a more intense workout or simply a bottle of water to sip on. Keep a post-workout snack nice and close as well—you may feel temporarily tired after your workout.

Gather your yoga mat or non-slip shower mat. Make sure any mat, socks, and shoes used are non-slip—you don't want to risk falling on your first attempt at Wall Pilates! Set up your music, if you're going to work out to a soundtrack.

Finally, take a look around and look for any potential safety habits. If you fell, where would you land? Is there anything hanging from the wall? Do you have your mobile device close enough to make a call? Preparing for the worst is better than hoping for the best when working out, so keep in mind that even though you're capable, accidents can happen.

Once your area is set up, you're ready to begin your workout in a safe, controlled environment, so let's get to it.

Chapter Two

Week 1: Building a Foundation

With everything set up, you're now ready to begin your Wall Pilates journey. Week 1 builds a solid foundation for your new exercise routine and eases you into some of the basic movements that will be built upon when progressing in your fitness and strength. Each of the movements in this chapter will help you form a strong base of Wall Pilates, prioritizing your safety and the inherent wisdom of your body.

We will begin the chapter with an introduction to basic movements moving on to your first set of core strengthening exercises. By starting with these elemental exercises, your body has the opportunity to become familiar with a new form of movement while you adjust to using the wall for support, balance, and resistance.

While some of these movements may seem somewhat rudimentary, they are more than a workout for your body. It's the beginning of a synergistic conversation your mind, body, and breath will be having to ensure you are building a mindful relationship with yourself. During these initial phases of your workout, make sure to become reflective and pay attention to what your body is telling you. Are you uncomfortable? Do you feel unbalanced? Can you feel your muscles engaging?

Mindful participation in your workouts will empower you, let you know where your limitations are, and will help you to understand when you're ready to move on to more challenging movements.

With the fundamentals and core workouts complete, you will move on to deep stretching. A round of stretching after a workout will minimize post-muscle stiffness, reduce your chance of injury, and release any residual tension in your muscles.

Finally, we will introduce you to breath techniques that can be used in your workouts for an added stress and anxiety-busting boost. While breathwork is a necessary part of your Wall Pilates workouts, these extra techniques can be used to complete a workout to calm your mind and body.

An Introduction to Basic Wall Pilates Movements

Before any workout, it's important to warm up your muscles with a series of target stretches that will reduce the risk of muscle strain and injury. These warm-up movements will also serve as the base upon which you will learn how to flow between movements rather than complete one stretch before moving on to another.

By the end of your final week of using Wall Pilates as a fitness companion, your goal should be to transition from one set of exercises to the next without taking a break. Having said that, this is not your goal right now. Instead, you're going to use your warm-up stretches as your movement tutor, training your body to breathe and flow through each different muscle stretch.

Warm-Up Stretches

Each of the stretches and movements below should be repeated 10 times, including individual limb exercises. This means you will need to complete 10 individual movements on one arm or leg before moving on to the other arm or leg.

Take your time when doing these warm-up movements. Concentrate on your breath and the precision of the movement rather than rushing through to get your warm-up done. We will begin at the top of your body, working your way down to your feet.

Neck and Shoulder Rolls

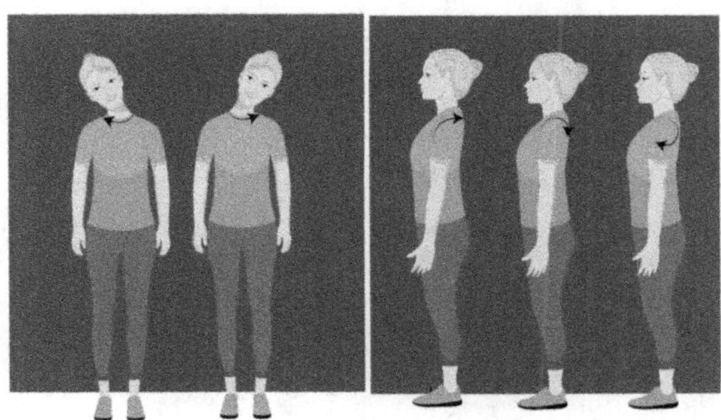

- Stand with your feet shoulder-width apart beside the wall. You can place the hand closest to the wall on the surface for additional support if you need it.

- Your free arm should be at your side.

- Take a deep breath in through your nose.

- As you exhale, gently lower your chin to your chest.

- Gently begin rolling your neck from the right to the back, then to the left, and finally, back to resting on your chest.

- Complete five full neck rolls.

- Repeat this movement in the opposite direction.

- Complete five full neck rolls.

- Return your head to a neutral position.

- If you're using the wall for support, let go and bring your hand and arm to your side.

- Begin rolling your shoulders in a circular motion from the front to the back.

- Complete five full forward rolls.

- Next, begin rolling your shoulders in a circular motion from the back to the front.

- Complete five full back rolls.

Arm Swings

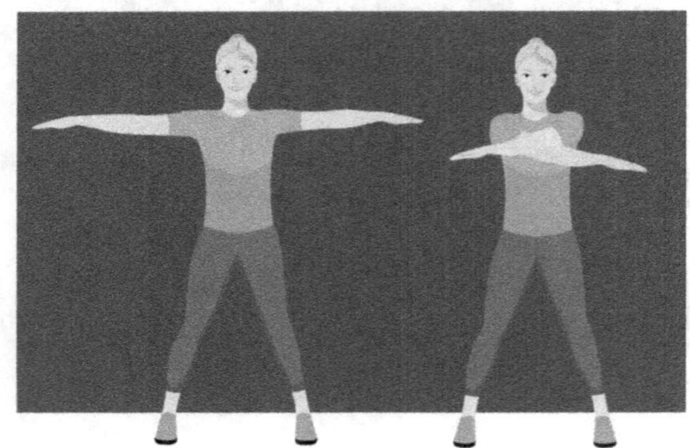

- Stand with your back to the wall and take one step forward to create about a foot's distance.

- Stand with your feet hip-width apart and make sure you're well-balanced.

- Extend your arms forward, keep them straight and parallel to the ground in front of you.

- Inhale deeply and as you do, move your arms outward until they're straight out at your sides, like airplane wings.

- Open and stretch your chest.

- As you exhale, bring your arms in front of you once more, crossing them slightly (but keeping them straight), at the wrist.

- Inhale once more and repeat this movement for 10 repetitions.

Wrist Rolls

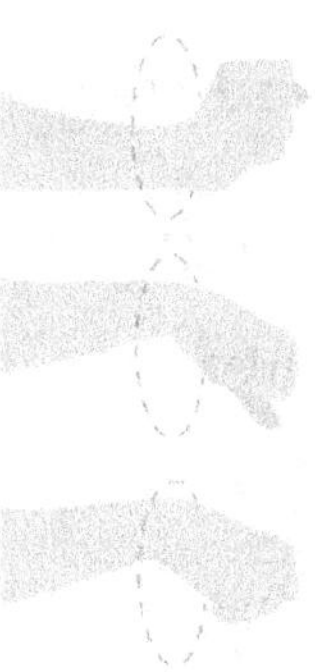

- Stand with your back against the wall, spine straight, and feet hip-width apart.

- Inhale slowly and lift your arms out in front of you.

- Try to keep your arms straight but do not lock your elbows.

- Begin to roll your wrists outwards and away from your body.

- Continue for five rolls, making sure to concentrate on your breath.

- Transition to inward wrist rolls, moving your hands inward toward each other.

- Continue for five rolls.

Hula Hoops

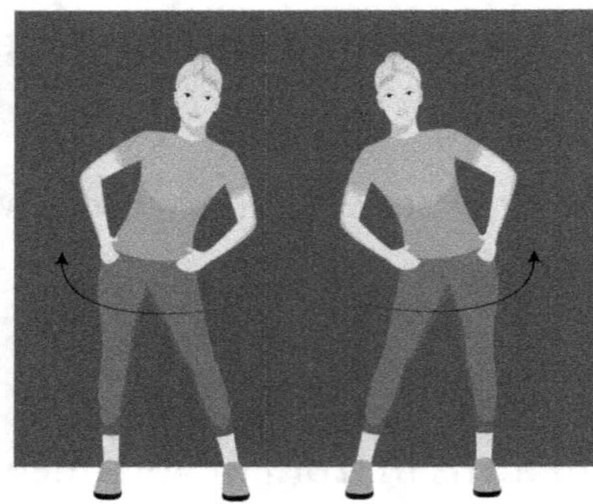

- Stand with your back to the wall and take one step forward to create about a foot's distance.

- Stand with your feet hip-width apart and make sure you're well-balanced.

- Place your hands on your hips and relax your shoulders.

- Bring focus to your breath and begin to roll your hips as if you were trying to keep a hula hoop spinning.

- Roll five times to the left and then switch directions, rolling five times to the right.

Leg Swings

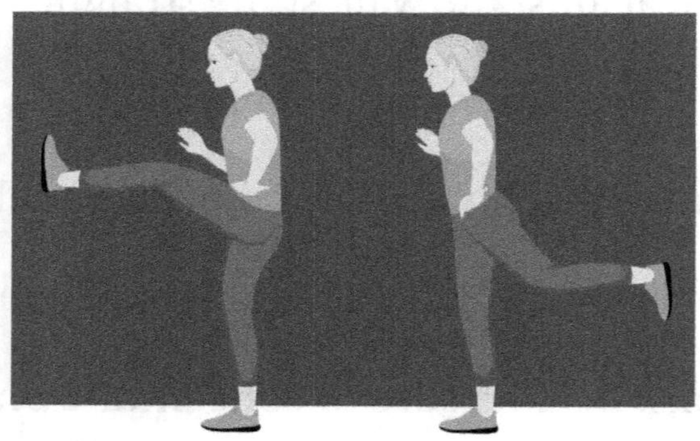

- Stand with your left side next to the wall.

- Extend your arm out and hold onto the wall for support.

- Bring focus to your posture, ensuring your spine is aligned and that your neck is relaxed.

- Lift your left leg (the one closest to the wall), and gently begin swinging it backward and forward.

- Make sure your movements are controlled and that you continue to breathe properly.

- Complete five full forward and backward swings.

- Place your left leg back on the floor and change position.

- Stand with your right side next to the wall.

- Extend your arm out and hold onto the wall for support.

- Bring focus to your posture, ensuring your spine is aligned and that your neck is relaxed.

- Lift your right leg (the one closest to the wall), and gently begin swinging it backward and forward.

- Make sure your movements are controlled and that you continue to breathe properly.

- Complete five full forward and backward swings.

- Place your right leg back on the floor and change position.

Ankle Rolls

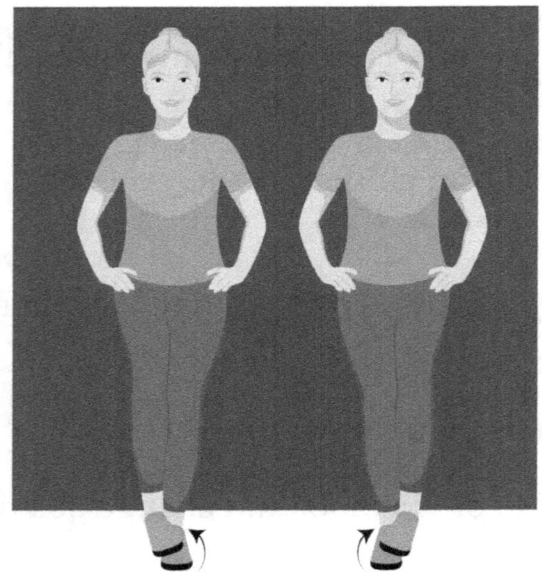

- Stand with your back against the wall, spine straight, and feet about hip-width apart.

- You can place the palms of your hands against the wall for additional support, or you can complete the exercise near a corner to ensure you feel supported.

- Lift your left leg up off the floor, just a few inches will do.

- Roll your foot at the ankle in whichever direction you're comfortable.

- Complete 10 left ankle rolls.

- Place your foot back on the floor.

- Make sure you are balanced and comfortable.

- Lift your right leg up off the floor, just a few inches will do.

- Roll your foot at the ankle in whichever direction you're comfortable.

- Complete 10 left ankle rolls.

- Place your foot back on the floor.

Foundational Workout

This first workout may seem short, sweet, and to the point but it is designed to challenge you as you transition into more robust workouts. With your first few attempts, take the time to pause between sets, checking in on your breathing, balance, and muscle comfort.

Once you have got the hang of the exercise, shorten your pause period or flow between each movement without a break. Remember that the goal of Wall Pilates is not to get a workout done, it's to slowly and carefully work through each movement, engaging your muscles, and focusing on creating a precise movement.

Wall Press

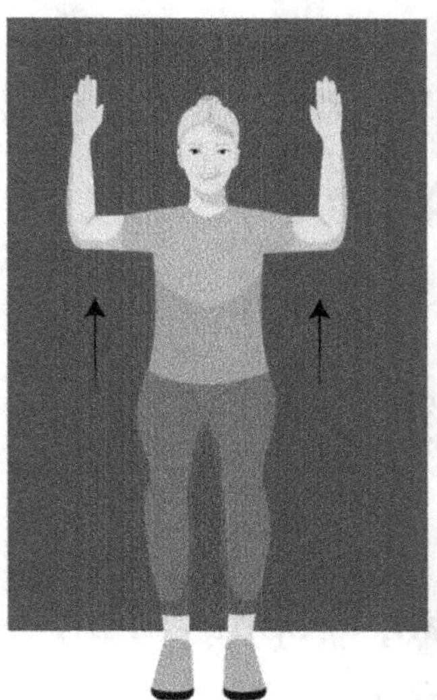

- Stand with your back to the wall.

- Your arms should be at your side, the backs of your hands pressed against the wall.

- Slide your arms up the wall, keeping them straight at the elbow and not lifting your hands off the wall.

- Once you reach a comfortable height, not more than shoulder height, gently press your arms against the wall.

- Hold for 5 full breath counts.

- Slowly slide your arms back down the wall to the starting position.

- Repeat this movement for 10 full repetitions.

Wall Slide

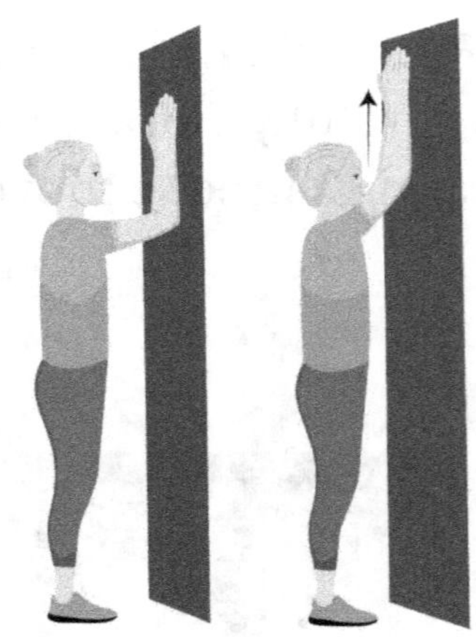

- Stand facing the wall.

- Place your arms on the wall with your hands side on with the wall (baby fingers against the wall.

- Slide your arms up the wall, keeping them slightly bent at the elbow and not lifting your hands off the wall.

- You should be creating a small circular motion with your arms, stopping just above shoulder height.

- Hold at your highest position for 3 full breath counts before slowly sliding your palms back down the wall to the starting position.

- Repeat this movement for 10 full repetitions.

Wall Squats

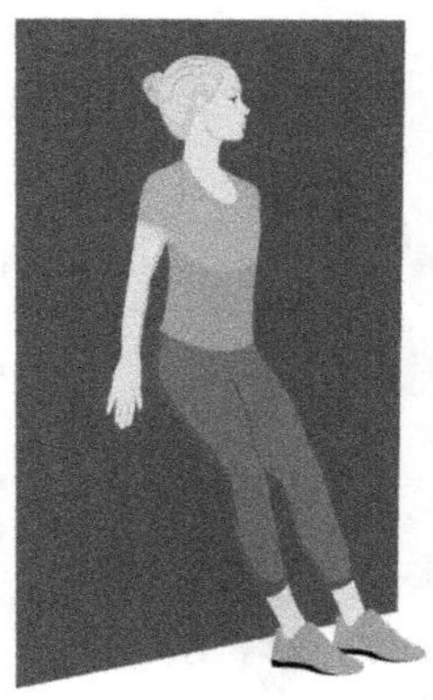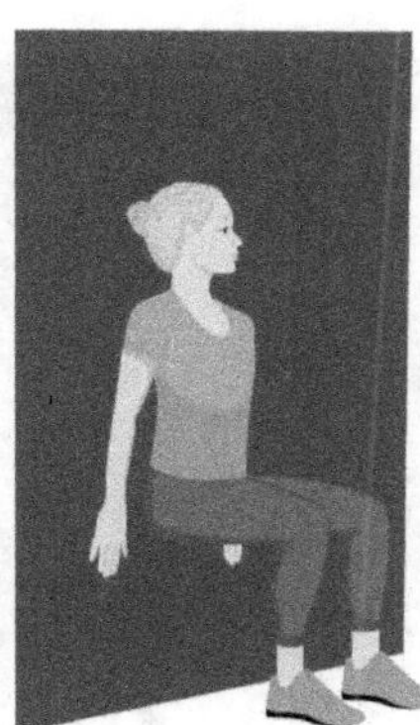

- Remain in your current position, back against the wall, feet shoulder-width apart.

- Place your palms against the wall for additional support, or on your hips if your legs are strong and can hold your weight when your knees are bent.

- Inhale deeply.

- As you exhale, slowly lower your body to the ground by bending your knees.

- Keep contact with your back and the wall.

- Once your thighs are parallel to the ground, hold your position for 3 full breath counts.

- If you are unable to go this low, stop where you are comfortable.

- Push through your heels, sliding back up the wall to your starting position.

- Repeat this movement 10 times.

Standing Wall Push

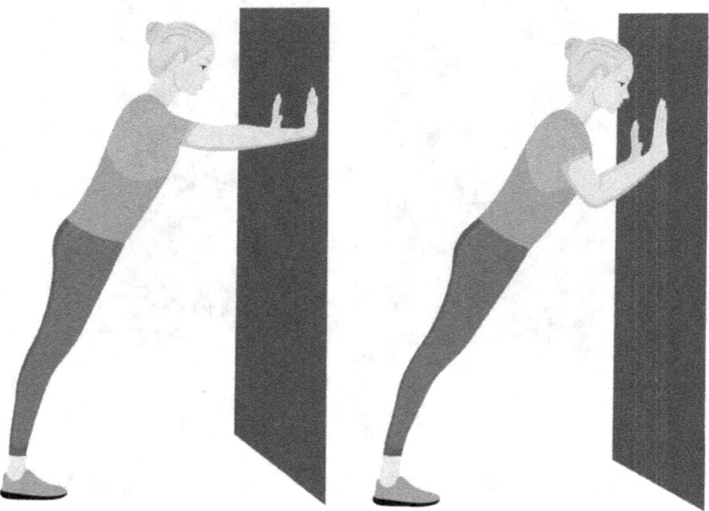

- Turn around and face the wall.

- Take a small step back so that you are about a foot's distance from the wall.

- Bring your arms out in front of you and place your palms against the wall.

- Inhale deeply.

- As you exhale, slowly and gently lower your body to the wall, bending your arms at the elbow.

- Hold your body weight in this bent position for three full breath counts.

- Push back through your arms, straightening your elbows so that you return to your starting position.

- Repeat this movement 10 times.

Wall Cat Stretch

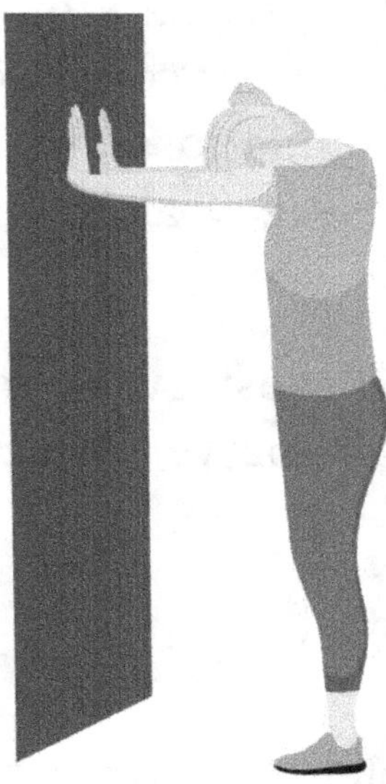

- Remain in your push-up position, facing the wall.

- Place your palms flat on the wall, fingers straight and pointing toward the ceiling.

- Lower your chin gently toward your chest, making sure to keep your neck relaxed.

- Inhale deeply and round your shoulders.

- Hold for three full breath counts and return to your starting position.

- Repeat for 10 full repetitions.

If you are not able to complete all repetitions, do as many as possible without discomfort. It's more important to draw focus to the rhythm between your movements and ensure you remain balanced and engaged. Keep in mind that it might take you slightly longer to feel comfortable with moving on to the more advanced techniques in Chapter 2. Wall Pilates is not a competition or a race, it's a personal journey to strength, mobility, and flexibility.

Core Strengthening Basics

A strong core is the essence of Wall Pilates and for good reason. Known as the body's central support system, strengthening your core goes beyond losing a couple of extra hormonal pounds. For many women, a loss of core strength after pregnancy can herald larger issues including back pain, weak hips, urinary incontinence, and pelvic dysfunction.

Because your core is integral to almost every motion you make, it's incredibly important in the management of pain, prevention of injury, and ensuring you remain poised and well-balanced.

Beginners Core Workout

Wall Pilates core exercises are completed on the floor, so make sure you have your grip mat or yoga mat at the ready.

Wall Sit-Ups

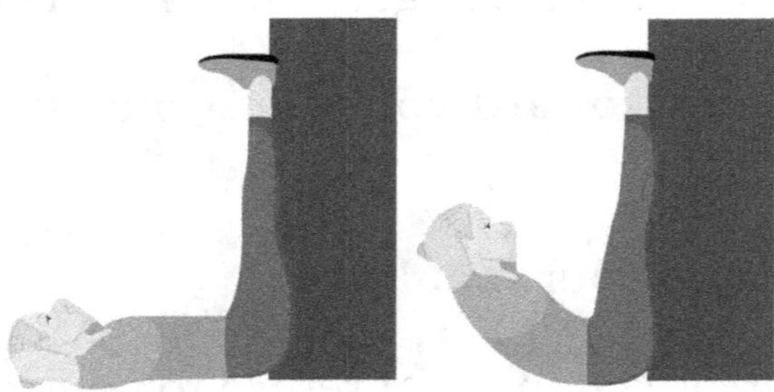

- Lie on the floor with your legs resting against the wall.

- Bend your knees slightly and open your feet about shoulder-width apart, placing them on the wall for more support.

- For stronger cores, cross your arms over your chest. For beginners, place your hands palms down on your thighs for additional support.

- To intensify your workout, keep your legs straight up against the wall.

- Inhale and engage your abdominal muscles.

- Lift your upper body toward your knees, bringing your shoulders in a curling motion.

- Make sure to keep your neck relaxed and don't hyperextend your upper back and shoulders.

- Slowly lower yourself down again.

- Repeat 10 times.

Wall Leg Pull-In

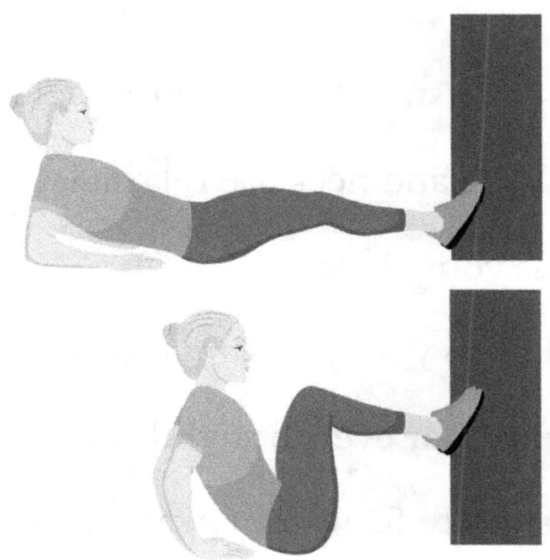

- Sit about a foot from the wall, back facing it.

- Place your hands behind you on the floor for balance.

- Lean back slightly and stretch your legs out.

- Lift your ankles off the floor ever so slightly.

- Inhale deeply.

- As you exhale, pull your knees toward your chest, contracting your abdominal muscles.

- Bring your legs down to the starting position immediately. Make sure your movements are controlled.

- Repeat for 10 full movement repetitions.

Wall Crunches

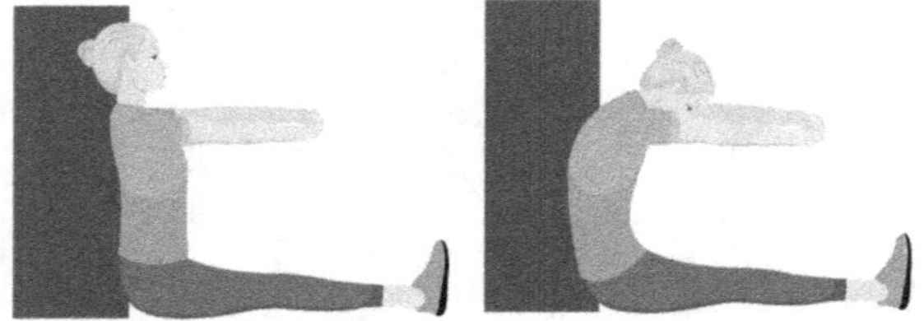

- Sit with your back flat and straight against the wall.

- Make sure your shoulders and neck are relaxed.

- Place your arms across your chest.

- Bend your knees and open your feet about shoulder-width apart.

- Lift your behind off the floor ever so slightly and make sure you are balanced.

- Roll your shoulders slightly forward, engaging your core, and crunching your abdominal muscles.

- Return to your start position.

- Repeat for 10 full repetitions.

Wall Bridge

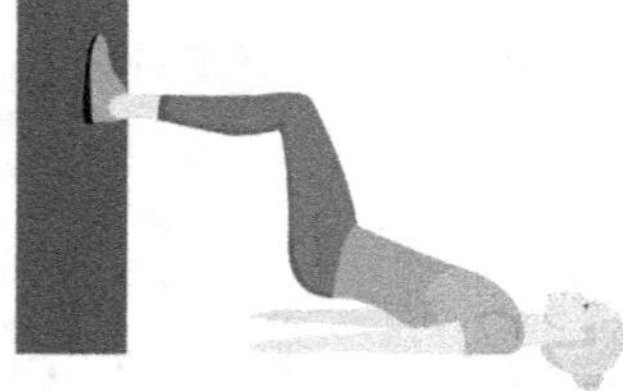

- Lie down on the floor, with your feet planted flat on the wall, knees slightly bent.

- Push your hips up, creating a straight line from your shoulders to your knees.

- Engage your abdominal muscles and focus on your breath.

- Hold this position for 5 full breath counts.

- Return to your starting position.

- Repeat this movement 10 times.

Wall Plank

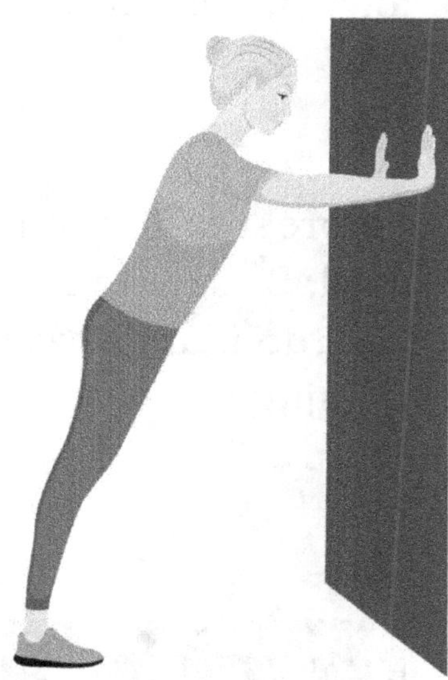

- Stand up and face the wall.

- Make sure your feet and mat are firmly planted and that you cannot slide.

- Take a big step back, putting about one and a half feet between you and the wall (you shouldn't be able to touch the wall).

- Gently lower your body forward, using your abdominal muscles to control your movement.

- Place your hands on the wall, bending your elbows slightly (you can lift yourself slightly onto your toes for more resistance if you like).

- Draw focus to your breath.

- Hold this position for ten full breath counts.

These core-centric exercises are essential for building the foundational strength you will need for more intensive Wall Pilates practices. By concentrating on progression, alignment, and gaining stability by engaging your core muscles, you're setting yourself up for a much stronger core.

Gentle Stretching for Flexibility: Cooling Down

Congratulations! Your first two workouts are now behind you! Cooling down and gentle stretching is a great way to end any workout. The movements in this section aren't just designed to minimize post-workout muscle stiffness but also to boost flexibility.

Flexibility Routine

As you age, your muscles become more stiff, and gentle stretching is a great way to keep your body agile and muscles relaxed. Be sure to move only as deep in these stretches as is comfortable for you. Don't overdo it and make sure that you are being mindful about your movements to prevent injury.

Wall Arm Slide

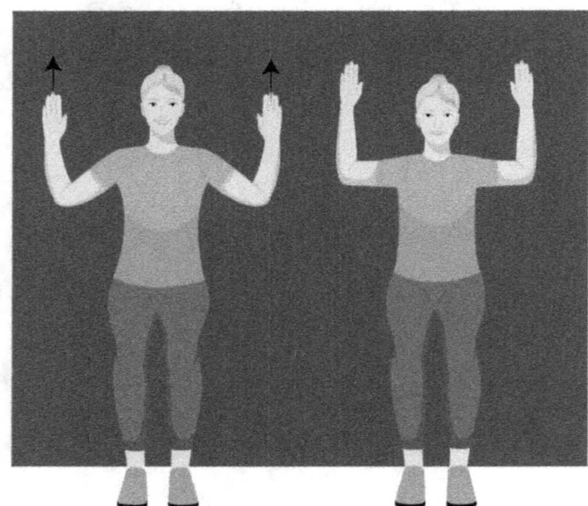

- Stand with your back gently resting against the wall.

- Extend your arms outward at shoulder height with elbows bent.

- Carefully slide your arms upwards, pressing softly against the wall.

- Hold your arms at shoulder height.

- Gently lift your shoulders off the wall, arching your back slightly.

- Hold this position for 10 full breath counts.

- Relax and return your shoulders to the wall and your arms to your side.

Wall Calf Stretch

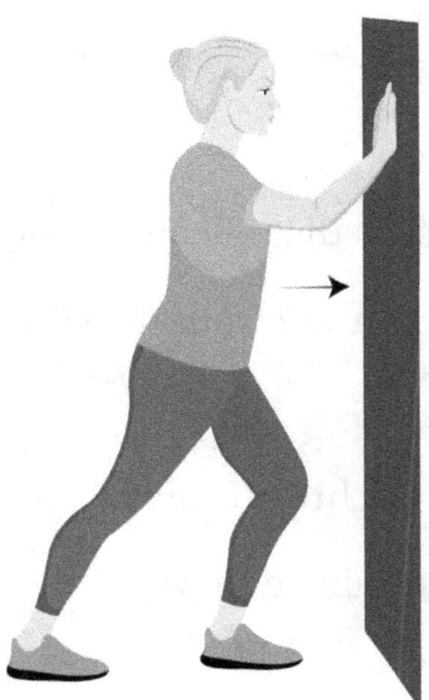

- Stand facing the wall.

- Take a small step back.

- Place your hands on the wall.

- Step back with one foot and gently press its heel downwards.

- Feel the stretch in the calf muscles as you press against the wall.

Wall Chest Opener

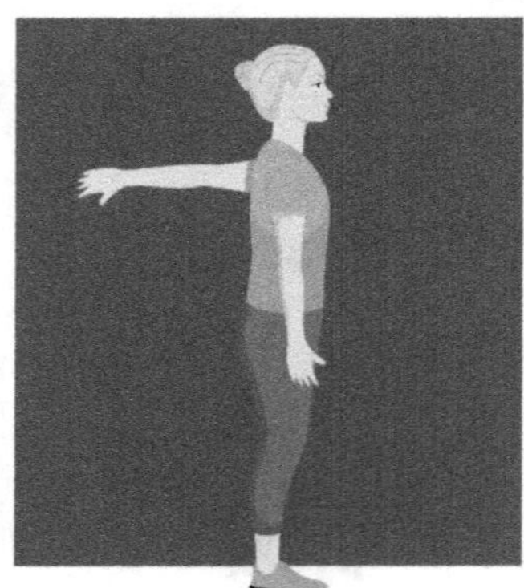

- Stand side-on to the wall.

- Straighten the arm closest to the wall and firmly place your hand against it.

- Gradually rotate your torso away from the wall, opening up the chest.

- Stretch pectoral muscles.

- Hold this position for 10 full breath counts.

- Switch sides and repeat the above steps.

Wall Hamstring Stretch

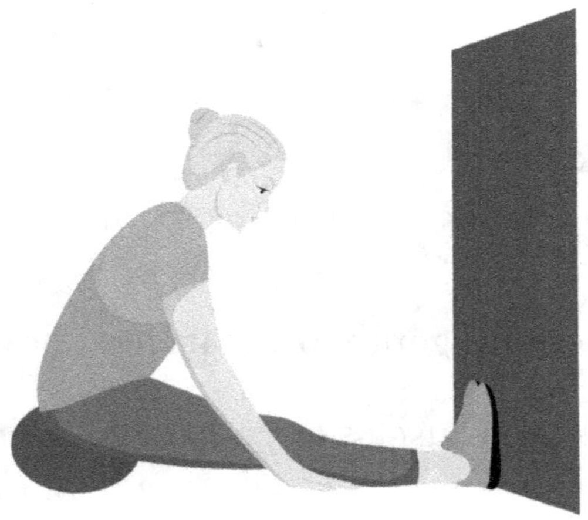

- Sit on the ground with your heels pushing gently against the wall.

- Keep your spine straight and inhale.

- Bring your arms up above your head and inhale.

- Bend your body forward, hinging at the hips and keeping your spine straight, reaching for the wall.

- Stop bending forward when you feel your hamstring stretch.

- Hold this position for 10 full breath counts.

Wall Butterfly Stretch

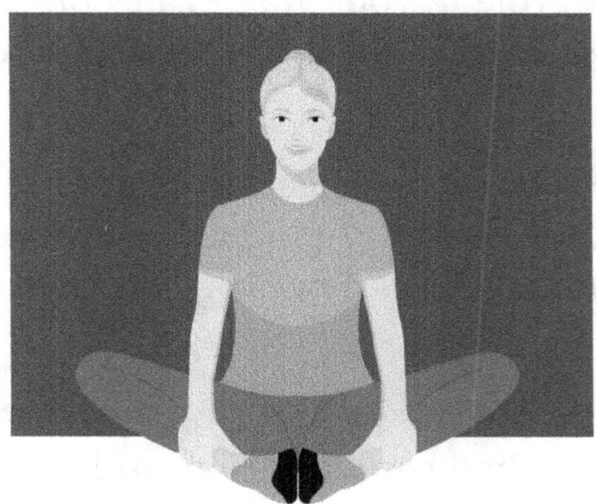

- Sit down with your back supported by the wall.

- Bring your knees up slightly, and press the soles of your feet together.

- Allow your knees to fall sideways.

- Lightly press down on your thighs with your elbows, deepening the stretch within your inner thigh and groin area.

- Don't overstretch, simply hold this position for 10 full breath counts.

Light stretching is a great way to learn flow between movements and can seriously boost the efficacy of your Wall Pilates workouts, elevating each workout to one that dynamically stretches and strengthens your muscles.

Each of the routines in this chapter are the very basics of Wall Pilates but will need to be perfected for you to move on to more challenging workouts and movements. While they may feel easy, try to increase your repetitions, making sure to build the strength and fluidity of your movements.

As your strength and flexibility increase, you'll require less recovery time and can spend more time perfecting your workouts.

Breathing Techniques for Wall Pilates

Breath plays a fundamental role in your Wall Pilates practice. Early on in your Wall Pilates practice, you may want to only focus on breathing adequately while you execute each move.

As you progress, however, you may feel like you want to change up your breathwork. Each of the breathing exercises below is designed to be worked into your Wall Pilates routine. Changes in breathing patterns, however, can cause some changes in the body including dizziness.

When incorporating new breathwork patterns into your Wall Pilates workout, be sure to pay close attention to your body and any signs of light-headedness. Alternatively, you can practice these techniques separately from your workouts until your body adjusts to different ways of breathing.

For Back Positions

- Position yourself with your back to the wall and feet planted a modest distance apart.

- Gently rest your hands over your abdomen.

- Draw in air slowly through your nostrils, allowing your belly to swell while keeping your chest's rise gradual and minimal.

- As you exhale, draw your belly inward, imagining the flow of air out of your mouth, like blowing through a straw.

- Repeat for 4 full breath counts, working your way up to 10 full breath counts.

For Rib and Shoulder Exercises

- Stand with your back resting against the wall and your hands on your ribs.

- Inhale deeply allowing your lungs to expand outward.

- Try to keep your belly contracted, minimizing its rise.

- On the exhale, pull your rib cage together, using your abdominal muscles to force the air out of your lungs.

- Repeat for 4 full breath counts, working your way up to 10 full breath counts.

For Stretching

- Sit with your spine against the wall and eyes closed.

- Inhale through your nose slowly, holding temporarily at your breath peak.

- Release the air slowly through pursed lips until your lungs feel empty.

- Repeat for 4 full breath counts, working your way up to 10 full breath counts.

Alternating days between your foundational workout, core workout, and dedicated stretching and breathwork will help even out your first week of Wall Pilates. Always remember to listen to your body, rest if your muscles are sore, and support your workouts with great nutrition and adequate hydration.

Chapter Three

Week 2: Enhancing Balance and Coordination

Week 2 moves you away from foundational exercise and gears your body toward the balance and coordination you will need to execute more advanced Wall Pilates movements. Each of the movements in this chapter is designed to precisely hone in on your body's stabilizer muscles and improve your overall balance.

Because balance is the cornerstone of your daily movement, it's important to work on maintaining equilibrium as a way to remain independent as you age. Coordination is, of course, the complementary counterpart to balance, helping you to perform daily movements with purpose and smoothly.

You will need balance to get just about anything done, from getting out of bed in the morning to hauling bags of groceries home, it's easy to forget that proper coordination and balance are required to maintain a good quality of life.

In this chapter, you're going to be introduced to targeted exercises that will not only build upon your existing foundation but challenge your body to remain in an upright position.

You may find that the intensity of your workouts begins to ramp up at this stage as new muscles are introduced to your Wall Pilates workout. Remember to honor your body and work at a pace that is sustainable for you. Use your breath to remain centered and grounded, and as you become stronger, begin to incorporate flow movements into your workouts.

Balanced-Focused Exercises

As we begin with week two, our focus shifts to more specialized muscle groups and more specifically, to the muscles that are required for a balance-centered lifestyle. This opening section is designed to bolster your balance, with an emphasis on the synergy between core strength and stability.

The essence of a strong core extends beyond superficial muscle development for a washboard stomach. Instead, it's the targeting of the deeper, stabilization muscles that are pivotal to posture and balance. Proprioception is your intrinsic ability to perceive your body's position and movement and a skill that can be honed through focused training. This in turn bolsters not just balance but the smoothness of your movement through daily life.

Each of the exercises listed in the workout below are specifically chosen to focus on strengthening your body's balance mechanisms and awakening the deep core muscles many of us neglect due to a lifetime of deskbound jobs. Over time, these exercises will build a network that supports daily movements and interactions to help maintain stability and fluidity in movement.

Balance-Focus Workout

You may want to choose to complete this workout near a corner or with additional support. While every care has been taken to ensure your safety while doing these exercises, it's important to note that they are designed to challenge your balance and poise. If additional support is not available in the form of a wall corner or other sturdy piece of furniture, consider having a friend present to ensure you remain safe and upright throughout your workout. You will also need a ball or pillow for this workout, so keep it handy and within arm's reach.

Wall-Mounted Tree Pose

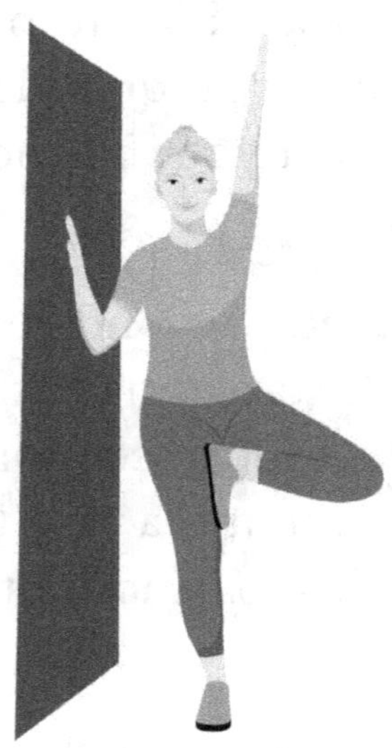

- Stand sidelong to the wall with one hand providing gentle support.

- Shift weight to one leg.

- Place one foot on the opposite inner thigh while standing tall—if you cannot reach your inner thigh, place your foot gently on your lower leg.

- Slowly raise the same arm as your lifted leg to the ceiling until it is straight.

- For a more challenging movement, try to lift your hand from the wall.

- Hold this position for 10 full breath counts.

- Shift sides, standing sidelong to the wall with your opposite side.

- Place one hand on the wall for gentle support.

- Shift weight to one leg.

- Place one foot on the opposite inner thigh while standing tall—if you cannot reach your inner thigh, place your foot gently on your lower leg.

- Hold this position for 10 full breath counts.

One-Legged Wall Squat Hold

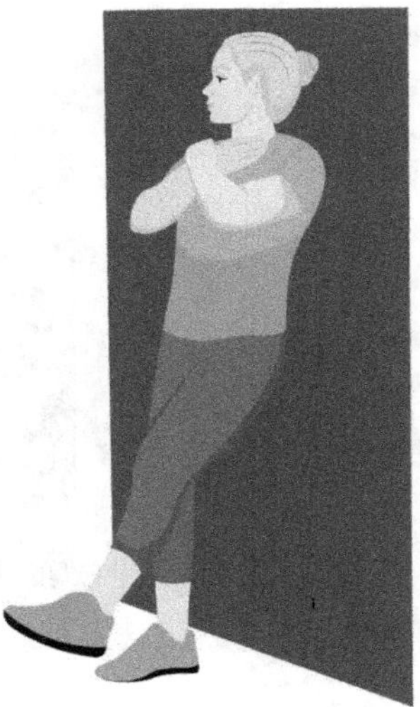

- Placing your back against the wall.

- Stand tall and make sure your spine is straight.

- Lift one leg off the floor.

- Bend your weight-bearing leg slightly at the knee—be sure to comfortably support your own weight and don't overextend yourself.

- Hold the position for 10 full breath counts.

- Return your foot to the floor.

- Lift the other leg off the floor.

- Bend your weight-bearing leg slightly at the knee—be sure to comfortably support your own weight and don't overextend yourself.

- Hold the position for 10 full breath counts.

Wall-Supported Leg Pulls

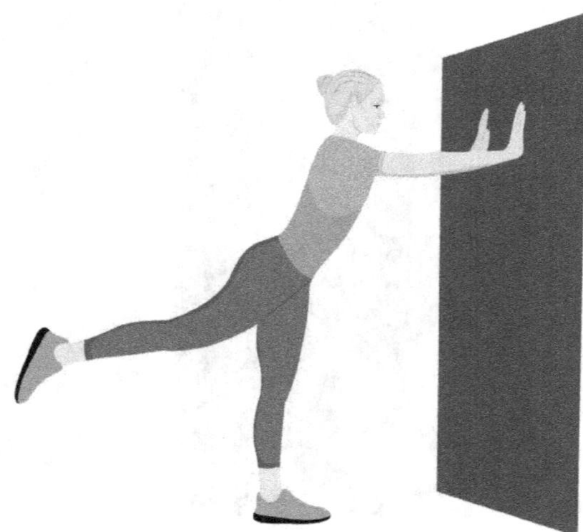

- Stand facing the wall with hands on the wall at shoulder height.

- Extend one leg behind you, keeping it lifted off the ground.

- Make sure you are balanced and that you're not using the wall for too much support. If you find you're using the wall too much, lower your lifted leg slightly.

- Hold this movement for 10 full breath counts.

- Return your foot to the floor.

- Now, extend your other leg behind you, keeping it lifted off the ground.

- Make sure you are balanced and that you're not using the wall for too much support.

- Hold this pose for 10 full breath counts.

Wall Stand and Squeeze

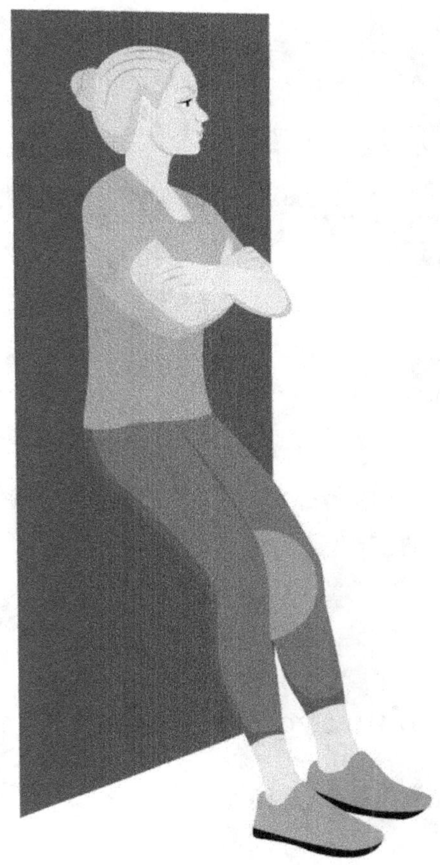

- Stand with your back to the wall, feet together.

- Place a ball or pillow between your knees so that it remains comfortably in position.

- Now, squeeze while maintaining an upright, balanced position.

- Hold the squeeze for 3 breath counts before releasing but ensure the pillow or ball doesn't fall to the ground.

- Repeat this movement 10 times.

Wall Supported Warrior III

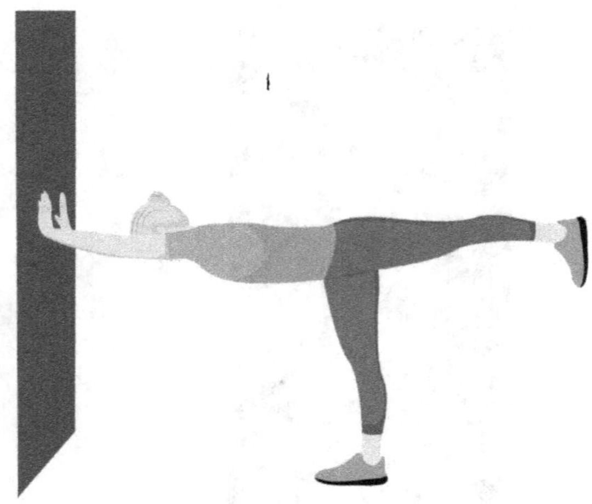

- Face the wall.

- Take a large step back so that you are about one and a half feet from the wall.

- Place your hands at shoulder height.

- Inhale deeply and as you exhale, extend one leg back.

- Lean forward as far as you can, stopping where you are comfortable or until your body forms a 'T' with the wall.

- Hold this position for 5 full breath counts.

- Replace your foot on the floor and stand upright.

- Now, extend the other leg back, leaning forward as far as you can.

- Hold this position for an additional 5 full breath counts.

End your workout with some light stretching to ensure you don't suffer from muscle stiffness the next day. Make sure to hydrate and eat a light snack as well. Remember, form is absolutely critical to any Wall Pilates workout so make sure to identify and address any imbalances you're experiencing before moving on to the next movement.

Coordinating Breath and Movement

Week 1 introduced you to fundamental breathing exercises. In week 2 we will begin to harmonize breath and movement, elevating your Wall Pilates stress-busting capabilities. While breathing properly throughout the course of a workout may seem simple enough, it is actually an art. If you tried the breathing techniques provided to you in Chapter 1, you would have soon come to realize that splitting your focus between movement and breath can be challenging.

If you begin to feel light-headed or dizzy at any point in these exercises, pause your workout, sit down, and wait for the feeling to pass before continuing.

Wall Angels

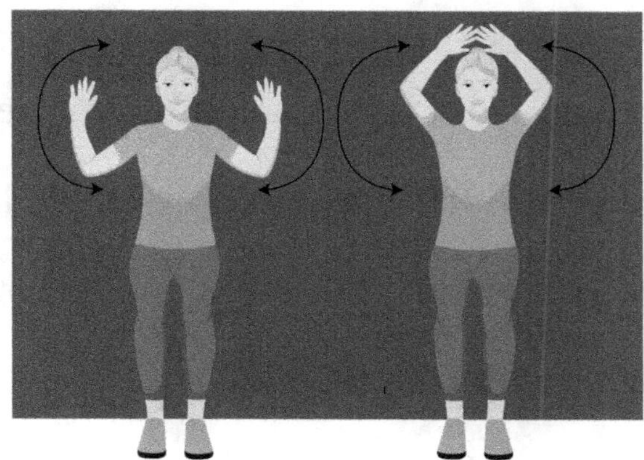

- Stand with your back against the wall, spine straight, and arms resting at your sides.

- Turn your palms out, away from the wall.

- Draw focus to your breath.

- Inhale deeply through your nose and as you do, begin to glide your arms up the wall, the backs of your hands touch at the peak of your breath.

- Pause your breath for a second before exhaling in a controlled manner through your mouth.

- As you exhale, bring your arms slowly back down to their starting position. Make sure that your arms and spine do not lose contact with the wall.

- Repeat this angel movement for 5 full breath counts, working your way up to 10 full breath counts.

Leg Ups With Breath

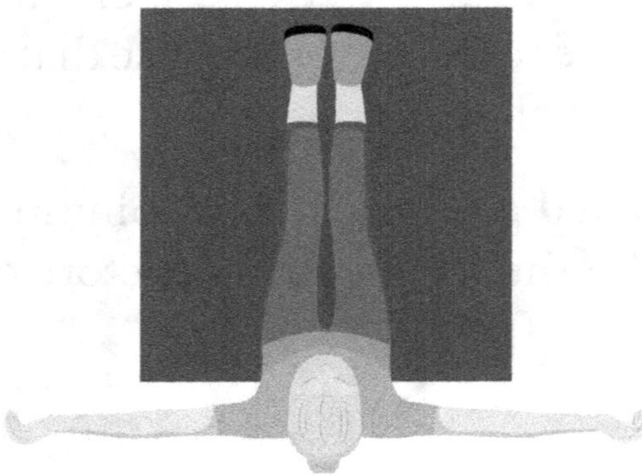

- Lay flat on your back with your legs straight up on the wall in front of you.

- Place your arms next to you for extra support, if you like.

- Alternatively, place one hand on your chest and the other on your belly.

- Inhale deeply through your nose, allowing your chest to rise but controlling the rise of your belly.

- Pause temporarily at the peak of your breath.

- Using your belly as the driving force, exhale through your mouth, and as you do, slowly lift your legs from the wall, holding them a few inches from it.

- Pause at the peak of your exhale.

- Now, inhale using your chest and slowly lower your back to the wall.

- Repeat this movement for 10 full breath counts.

Hip Opening Core Crunch

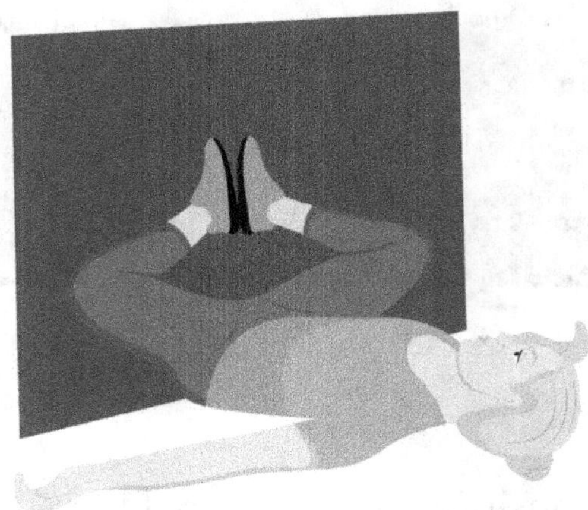

- Lay flat on your back with your legs straight up on the wall in front of you.

- Place your arms next to you for extra support.

- Slowly lower your legs down the wall until your feet comfortably touch in a butterfly position.

- You can shift your behind closer to the wall for a deeper stretch if this position is too easy for you.

- Slowly inhale through your nose, pausing at the peak of your breath.

- As you exhale, gently lift your shoulders off the floor, crunching your abdominal muscles.

- Hold this position as you pause on your exhale.

- Slowly lower your shoulders back to the floor as you inhale slowly.

- Repeat this movement for 10 full breaths.

- **NOTE: During your upward, exhale movement, be sure to keep your neck and shoulders relaxed. If you feel any strain in your neck, reposition your body into a more relaxed stance and try again.**

Breath Pulse Squats

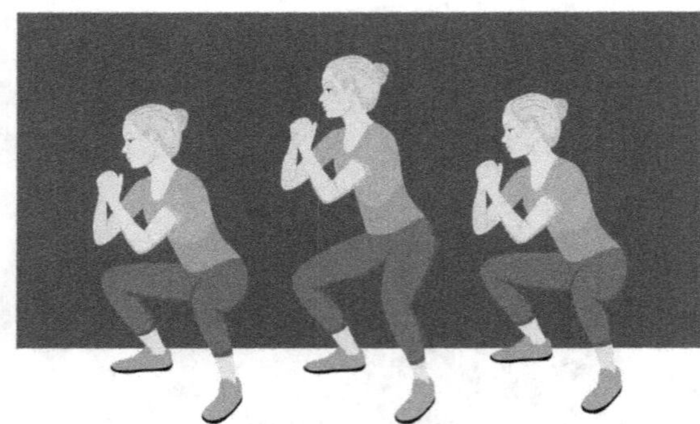

- Return to a standing position carefully, making sure that you are not too dizzy and that you are supported.

- Stand with your back against the wall, feet about shoulder-width apart.

- Place the palms of your hands on your thighs for additional support.

- Inhale through your nose slowly and as you do, slowly begin to lower your body into a comfortable squat position.

- At the peak of your inhale, pause for a moment.

- Now, begin to exhale through your mouth and as you do, pulse gently up and down.

- For a more advanced movement, time your outward breath with each pulse, pausing on the up-pulse and exhaling with the down-pulse.

Standing Oblique With Breath

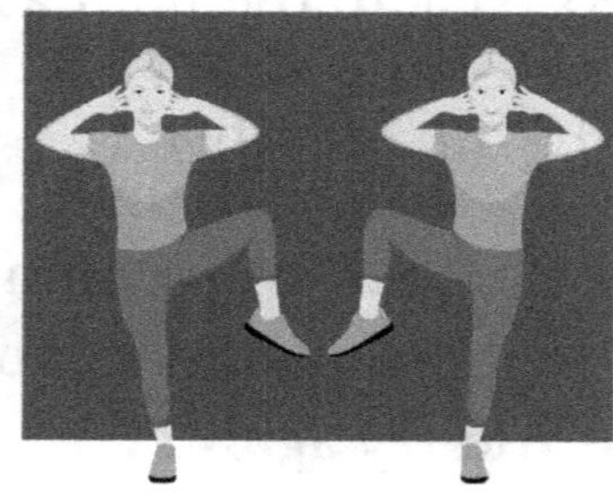

- Stand with your back toward the wall, with a small gap between your body and it.

- Lift your arms up and rest your palms behind your head, elbows parallel to the floor.

- Inhale slowly through your nose and as you do, lift your leg, knee bent at a 90% angle, up toward your hips.

- At the same time, drop the same elbow down to meet with your knee, crunching your obliques on that side.

- Exhale through your mouth slowly as you return your foot to the floor and your elbow to the starting position.

- Complete 5 of these movements on one side.

- Switch sides and make sure you are balanced.

- Lift your arms up and rest your palms behind your head, elbows parallel to the floor.

- Inhale slowly through your nose and as you do, lift your opposite leg, knee bent at a 90% angle, up toward your hips.

- At the same time, drop the same elbow down to meet with your knee, crunching your obliques on that side.

- Exhale through your mouth slowly as you return your foot to the floor and your elbow to the starting position.

- Complete 5 of these movements on this side.

These breath and movement exercises may be challenging so don't worry if your coordination isn't quite where you'd like it to be. Place more focus on your safety and perfecting these moves so that they become second nature and you find yourself automatically controlling your breath while completing any workout.

Building Posture and Alignment

Proper posture supports your balance and helps keep your muscles and bones aligned for a pain-free life. This section's workouts are aimed at strengthening posture awareness, enhancing overall alignment, and correcting any disparities in form you may have.

For many of us, entering into our 50s comes with a profound awareness that we have neglected our strength and posture in our younger days. Backaches, sore shoulders, and muscle stiffness hinder our movements and pain can contribute to lowered mood. The exercises in this portion of your workout routine are not just straightening up your stance though, they're meant to help you become more in tune with your body's natural alignment so that you can begin to build strong muscles that counteract muscle pain and strains.

Posture and Poise Routine

Wall Posture Check

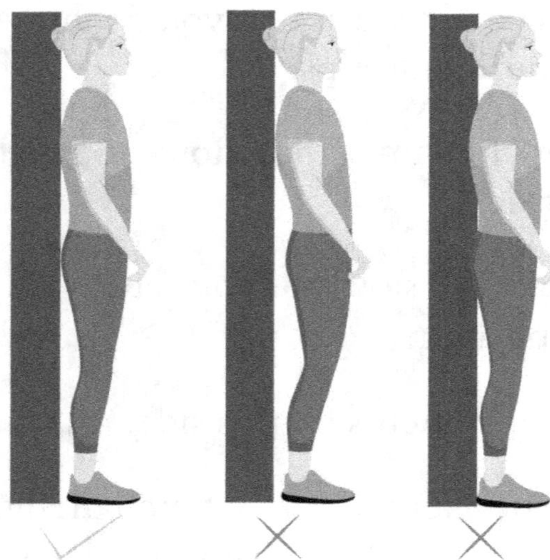

- Stand with your back to the wall, against it.

- Take a moment to mindfully scan your body. What areas of your body naturally touch?

- Assess which areas of your body are not touching the wall—your buttocks, shoulders, and the back of your head should be in light contact, with a small natural curve in your lower back.

- Readjust your position until each of the touching areas mentioned above is in light contact with the wall.

Wall Pelvic Tilt

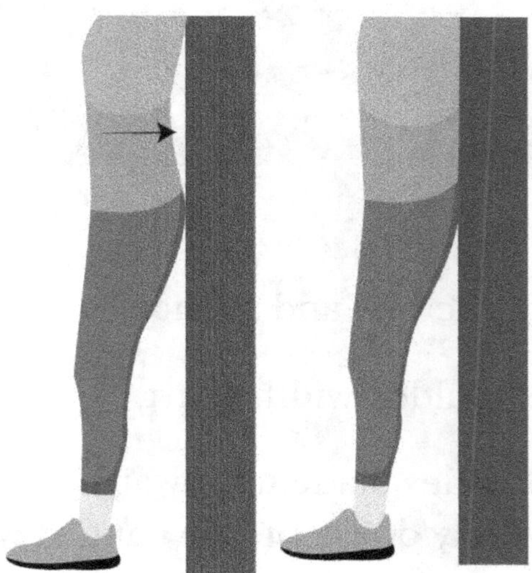

- From your starting Posture Check position, take a small step forward, placing about half a foot distance between the wall and your heels.

- Lean your body back until your behind, spine, shoulders, and back of your head are making contact with the wall.

- Bring your arms up to shoulder height, straight out next to you, and make contact with the wall (palms facing inward).

- Now, gently arch the center of your spine, making sure the small of your back is not in contact with the wall but your behind, shoulders, and head remain in contact—tilt your pelvis.

- Hold this position for 3 breath counts.

- Relax and flatten your entire spine against the wall again.

- Repeat this movement 10 times.

Wall Scapula Slide

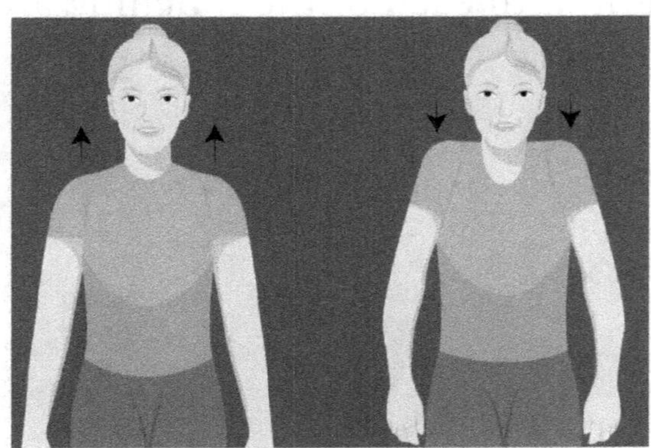

- Stand with your back to the wall and anchor your spine to it.

- Open your feet about shoulder-width apart.

- Now, slide your left shoulder blade up toward your ear in a shrugging motion, making sure that your body does not lose contact with the wall.

- Hold the position for 3 breath counts and return to your neutral position.

- Lift your right shoulder blade up toward your ear in a shrugging motion.

- Hold the position for 3 breath counts and return to your neutral position.

- Complete 5 repetitions per shoulder (10 repetitions in total).

As you move through these exercises, use the wall as more of a guide and less for support. This will allow you to gently adjust your body's positioning. While these movements may not have you breaking into a sweat, they do ensure your posture is corrected over time, improving your balance, realigning your muscles, and perfecting your Wall Pilates form for maximum impact.

Progress Tracking and Adaptation

Before venturing into your next week's Wall Pilates workouts, it's important that you know how to track your progress and adapt your workouts. Meticulous observation of your Wall Pilates progress serves two purposes—to have a tangible record of where you started and how you've progressed, and the ability to carefully analyze your workouts so that you can tweak movements where you need to.

As you begin to progress into the more challenging workouts in upcoming chapters, you may begin to notice that certain areas of your body are improving faster than others. This is perfectly normal, especially for women who tend to have more leg strength and coordination and less core strength. A number of factors come into play when it comes to building strength including your previous levels of strength and fitness, pregnancies, abdominal surgeries, the nature of your job, and how active you are now.

Charting your progress provides you with a visual representation of your changing body and allows for ongoing refinement when it comes to your personal strength, flexibility, and balance needs. No two bodies are built the same and no two bodies will respond to Wall Pilates in the same way. Noticing patterns in your advancement allows you to place more focus on one area of development while still working out your body as a whole.

This final section of our Balance and Coordination chapter provides you with the tools you need to adequately track your progress and a free gift that will elevate your Wall Pilates journey.

Tools to Track Your Progress

From good old pen-and-paper journals to modern apps, tracking your progress at home has never been easier. Aside from these two means, however, you can test your increasing levels of strength with some at-home tools and tricks.

1. Begin by setting yourself a goal. Do you want to become stronger, more flexible, improve your balance, or reduce your pain? Providing yourself with just one wellness goal at a time will help you feel less overwhelmed about all of the work you feel like you need to do to improve. Break each of these goals down into smaller milestones—like 10 minutes of Wall Pilates daily—to help you keep focused and on track with your overall goal.

2. Keep your goals overarching by remaining focused. The days of dramatic dieting and trying to live up to society's body standards are now long gone. This is a good thing because you can begin to focus on overarching goals that are

important to you. If your main goal is to build more muscle strength, apply an overarching goal of increasing protein in your diet to support lean, strong muscle development.

3. Embrace resistance as a matter of urgency. Wall Pilates is, by nature, a form of resistance exercise, but this doesn't mean you cannot add more resistance to your workouts. As you progress and become stronger, consider adding tools like resistance bands to your workout so that you can ramp up the intensity of your exercise without having to lift clunky weights.

4. Be as consistent with your tracking as you are with your workouts but don't obsess. Your body is going to ebb and flow throughout your fitness journey. There will be times when you're too stiff to do a proper workout and times when you feel like you've made no progress at all. Consistent tracking shows you how far you've come with your workouts and lets you know that you are way better off than when you first started.

5. Listen to your body at all times. If something is hurting or you don't feel like you're strong enough for an intense workout, give it a skip, opting for gentle stretching or deep breathing for that day. Overexerting your body is only going to set you back on your fitness journey and no one wants to be nursing an injury when they could be getting strong and lean.

Chapter Four

Week 3: Alleviating Back Pain and Strengthening Joints

Getting older often comes with aches and pains we didn't experience when we were older. For a lot of women, aching joints and lower back pain can deter us from adequate physical movement. The good news is that Wall Pilates exercises are specifically designed to tackle discomfort and improve the functional capability of our bodies.

Throughout this chapter, you will be introduced to movements that are meant to soften the grips of back pain and amplify the resilience of your joints through careful, targeted routines. While life's normal wears and tears can't really be undone, we can build an exercise routine that will help to slow down any additional issues as well as strengthen our muscles so that we can overcome pain.

Much of the emphasis of these workouts will focus on the physical action required to strengthen each of your poses, recalibrate the balance, and stretch your aching muscles in an effective way. Remember, Pilates is a preferred rehabilitation exercise that is used by millions the world over to provide lasting comfort and an expanded range of movement. Healthcare professionals and physiotherapists endorse Wall Pilates as a balanced approach to improving health and well-being but it is up to you to control your movements, work within your limitations, and be purposeful in the execution of each of your movements.

Back Pain Relief Exercises and Strengthening Exercises

This workout shifts our attention toward exercises, tailored for Wall Pilates and that offer respite from back pain. Each of these exercises is constructed with careful consideration for your back's health and the overall health of your spine.

I know all too well how debilitating back pain can be and how it impedes physical activity and the general quality of your life. In the beginning phases of Wall Pilates, one of my primary concerns was focused on how I was going to manage my back pain after completing a workout.

I quickly discovered that if I spent more time focusing on the deepness of each stress and movement and less time worrying about getting through the workout or my physical limitations, Wall Pilates actually reduced my chronic pain.

Of course, these results weren't immediate, but over time, I noticed considerably less pain and a much greater range of motion. The same will be true for you, so be patient, work on your form, and pretty soon, you'll realize you're doing a lot more than you used to without as much pain.

Back Pain Relief Workout

You will need a non-slip mat and a rolled-up towel or foam roller to support your lower back during this workout. If you feel like you don't need additional support at this stage, feel free to leave your towel or roller to one side.

Pelvic Curl Against the Wall

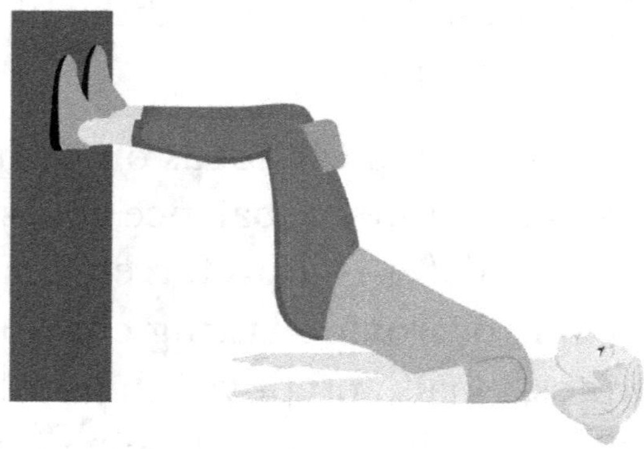

- Lie down on your back, facing the wall.

- Bring your feet up and press them against the wall about hip-width apart.

- Scoot your behind a little closer to the wall if necessary so that your knees are slightly bent.

- Engage your core and inhale deeply.

- On your exhale, raise your hips off the floor using your glutes and abdominal muscles to control the movement—this should be a tilting, not a thrusting movement.

- As you inhale, slowly lower your pelvis back to the floor.

- For a deeper stretch, grip your foam roller or towel between your knees, squeezing it on your upward movement.

- Repeat this movement 10 times.

Wall-Supported Knee Rolls

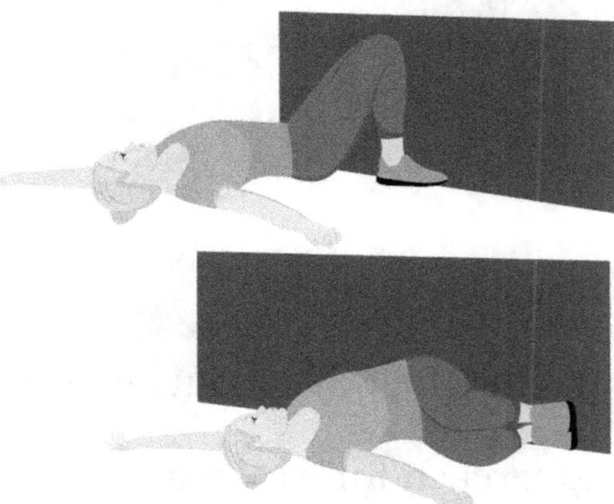

- Remain in your Pelvic Curl position, but move slightly further away from the wall so that only your toes make contact with it.

- Remove your towel or roller if you are using one.

- Place your arms out parallel to the wall and palms on the floor for extra stability.

- Gently rotate your knees to the left, rolling at the hip.

- Hold this position for 2 breath counts.

- Return to your center position.

- Now, gently rotate your knees to the right, rolling at the hip.

- Hold this position for 2 breath counts.

- Return to your center position.

- Complete 5 rolls per side—10 in total.

Wall Child's Pose

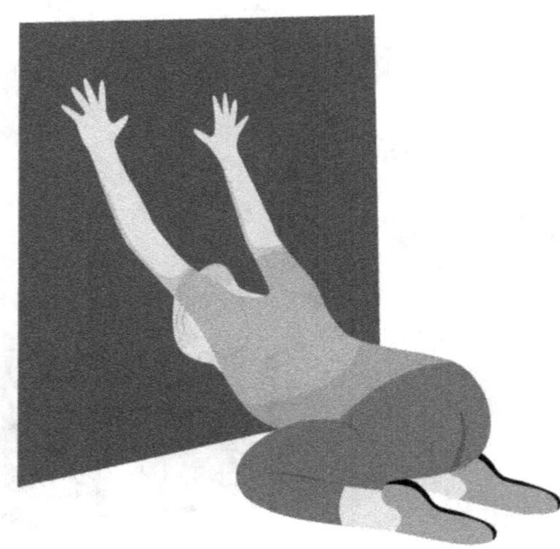

- Sit up on your knees, facing the wall, about an arm's length away.

- In this kneeling position, reach forward with straight arms and place the palms of your hands on the wall—the lower your arms, the deeper the stretch so begin with your arms higher up the wall and test your pain level.

- Inhale and slowly press your arms against the wall, stretching and elongating your spine.

- Stop when you feel the stretch and hold for ten full breath counts.

- Return to your starting position.

Wall Spine Straightener

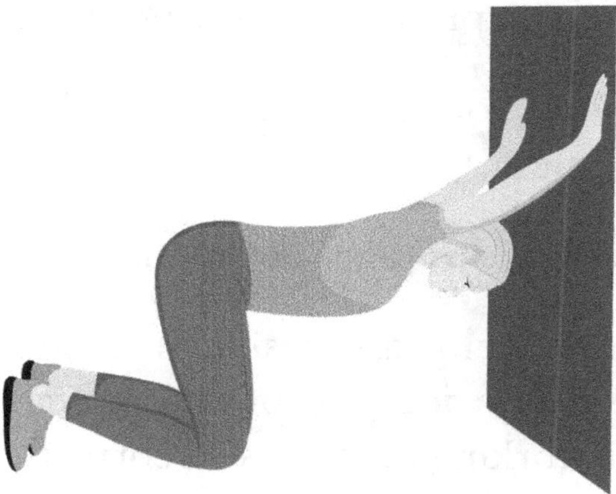

- Remain in your Child's Pose position.

- Place your hands on the wall, directly in front of you so that your arms are parallel to the floor.

- Ensure your palms are flat on the wall and you have enough grip.

- Slowly begin lifting your body up at the knees until your spine is straight and your knees are at a 90-degree angle—you should look like a tabletop.

- Keep your spine straight with as little pressure as possible on your arms and hands.

- Hold this position for 10 full breath counts.

Wall Push-Offs

- Carefully rise to a standing position.

- Continue to stand and face the wall.

- Position your hands on the wall, about shoulder height—your palms need to be flat on the wall and your arms straight but elbows should not be locked.

- Take a deep breath and lower your body to the wall by bending your elbows—as if you were doing a push-up against the wall.

- As you exhale, push your body away from the wall in a fluid, controlled movement.

- Your aim is to return to an upright, standing position without the aid of the wall.

- Inhale once more, and as you exhale, push your body away from the wall in a fluid, controlled movement.

- Complete 10 full repetitions of this movement.

Keep in mind that these movements are designed to be implemented with precise execution. It's better to focus on the deepness of your stretches so that the right muscles are engaging and that you're working each muscle correctly.

Joint-Specific Movements for Mobility

Exercises that are designed specifically to target and boost joint mobility, prevent injury, and reduce muscle stiffness are absolutely essential as we age. While our range of movement certainly does reduce as we get older, it's important to place focus on enhancing flexibility so that we can expand our range of motion. Added to this, the joints that often restrict our movements because of pain or a lack of flexibility, are the ones we need to be able to move more fluidly through life. In targeting these joints with proper exercise, you can reclaim not only your flexibility and ease of movement but also your confidence as you begin to move with more confidence.

Joint-Specific Workout

When working through this routine, make sure to center yourself and engage your core muscles for additional stability. Be safe in your practices and don't overextend your joints. Instead, pause at the height of each movement, choosing to hold the stretch in place. As you progress through your workouts, there will be plenty of time to test your limits and work on intensifying your workouts.

Wall Figure of Four

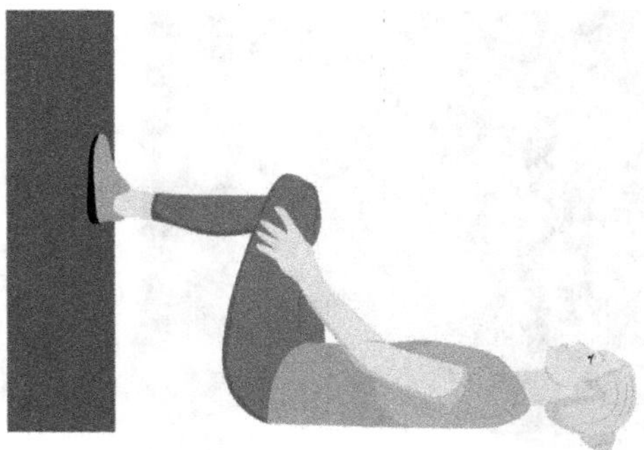

- Lie on your back with your behind facing the wall.

- Place your feet flat on the wall and make sure your knees are slightly bent.

- Place your hands at your sides on the floor or on your legs for additional support.

- Lift one leg off the wall, bending it at the knee.

- Rest the ankle of your bent leg on the opposite knee.

- Try to extend your hip out toward the floor.

- Hold this position, while controlling your breath for 5 full breath counts.

- Return your bent leg to its original position.

- Restabilize your body.

- Complete this movement with the opposite leg, holding for 5 full breath counts.

- Return your bent leg to its original position.

Wall Scissors

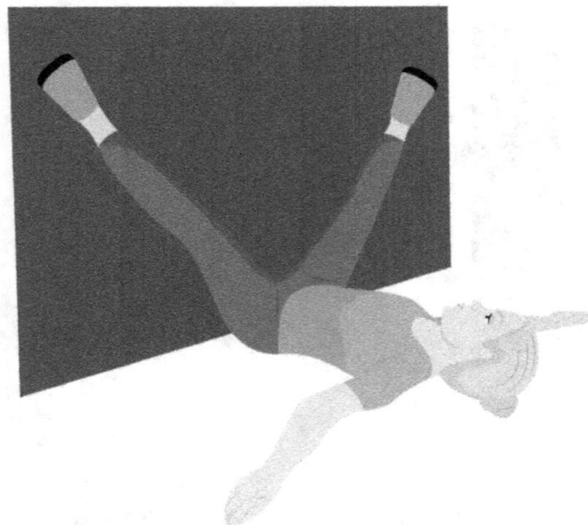

- Remain lying on the floor.

- Lift your legs straight up against the wall, shifting your behind until you can keep your legs comfortably stretched but straight at the knee.

- Place your arms on the floor, spread out and your palms facing down so that you remain balanced.

- Inhale deeply.

- On your exhale, open your legs in a controlled movement—a scissors motion. Keep your movements controlled and slow.

- Return your legs to a closed position as you exhale.

- Repeat this movement 10 times.

Leg Circles

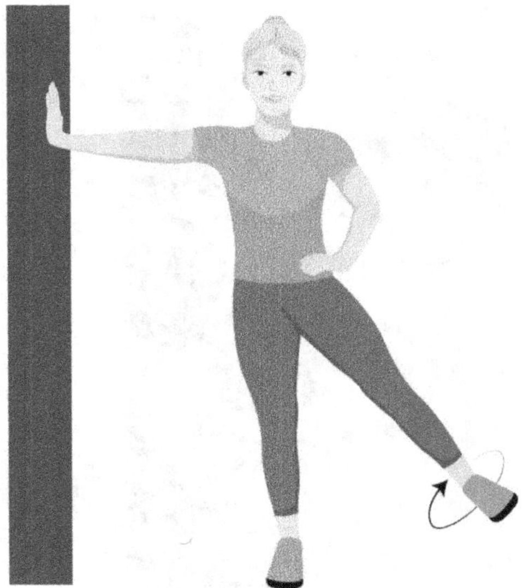

- Stand up slowly, using the wall for support.

- Stand side on to the wall with your left arm extended out.

- Place your palm flat against the wall and make sure your supporting arm is straight but the elbow isn't bent.

- Place your right hand on your hip for extra balance.

- Next, slowly lift your right leg off the floor, making sure your leg remains straight.

- Complete 10 circular movements with your lifted leg, alternating between front and back.

- Place your leg back on the floor.

- Switch sides with your right palm using the wall for support.

- This time, lift your left leg off the floor, making sure your leg remains straight.

- Complete 10 circular movements with your lifted leg, alternating between front and back.

- Place your leg back on the floor.

Wall-Supported Cobra Pose

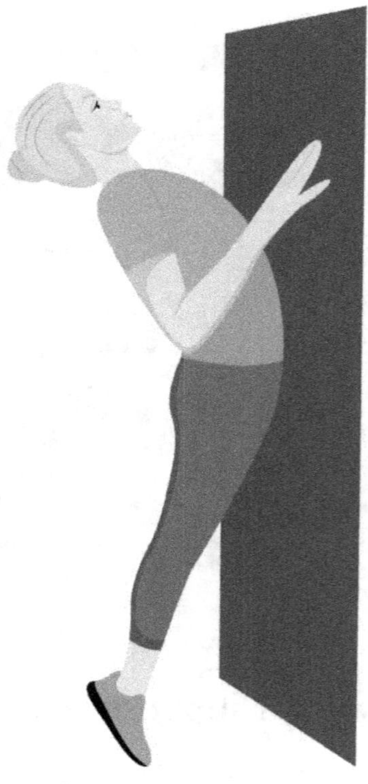

- Shift closer to the wall and face it—you should be about a foot away.

- Place your palms on the wall at about chest height, elbows bent, and to your sides.

- Inhale deeply.

- On your exhale, arch your lower back with the aim of lifting your chest off the wall and making contact with your pelvis.

- To deepen the stretch, you can stand on your toes—this challenges your balance so be careful.

- Hold this pose for 5 full breath counts.

- Return to a neutral standing position, standing still and focused for 5 full breath counts.

- Repeat this movement one more time.

Chest and Shoulder Mobility Stretch

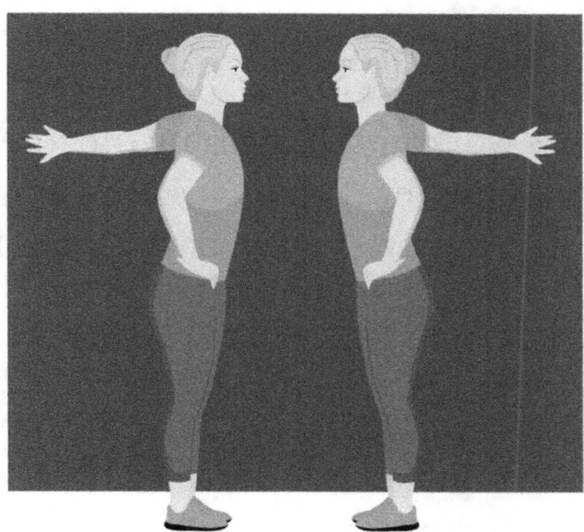

- Return to a side on position to the wall.

- Extend your arm out to the side and place your palm flat on the wall.

- Your arm should be straight but your elbow should not be locked.

- Keeping your hand in place, begin to rotate your body toward the front-facing position.

- When the stretch is deep but comfortable, pause and hold for 5 full breath counts.

- Return to your starting position, extending your arm out to the side and placing your palm flat on the wall.

- Your arm should be straight but your elbow should not be locked.

- Keeping your hand in place, begin to rotate your body toward the front-facing position.

- When the stretch is deep but comfortable, pause and hold for 5 full breath counts

Weaving these specialized joint exercises into your Wall Pilates routine promotes flexibility, soothes joint pain, and improves overall mobility. Over time, each of these movements can be interwoven into longer, more intensive Wall Pilates workouts, greatly improving how dynamic your workouts can be.

Intermediate Core Strengthening

It's time to ramp up your core workouts, increasing the intensity of your foundational core exercises to an intermediate level. This will challenge your stability, enhance spinal support, and burn any unwanted pounds you may have accumulated around the midriff.

The exercises in this workout connect the initial movements you've mastered with more advanced and intensive exercises. This promotes a steady and effective progression through your Wall Pilates journey. Remember, your core is central to your balance, and is essential for sustaining posture and in facilitating proper daily movement. Improving your core strength is vital to maintaining equilibrium and stability and burning away any pesky pounds that may be hanging on.

Intermediate Core Workout

You may need a pillow or rolled-up towel to support your hips and lower back during these exercises. Make sure you have either of these on hand so that you don't have to pause your workout. Added to this, you will be spending some time on the floor, so ensure your non-slip yoga mat is laid out in your workout space.

Controlled Leg Extensions

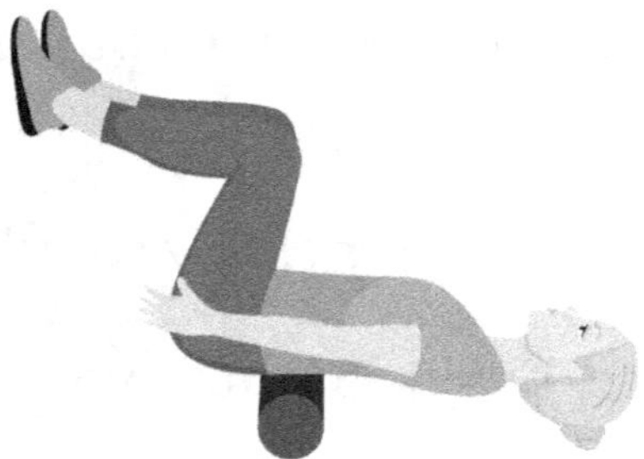

- Lie on the floor with your head against it.

- You can place a cushion or rolled-up towel under your behind to intensify your workout.

- Place your hands on the floor next to you for extra support. Alternatively, place your hands on your belly or the pillow/towel to intensify your workout.

- Now, inhale and elevate your hips off the floor, lifting your legs above your head.

- Make sure to bend at the hips and use your core muscles to execute the movement.

- On your exhale, slowly lower your legs to the floor, using your abdominal muscles to control the movement.

- Repeat 10 full movements.

Intermediate Wall Plank

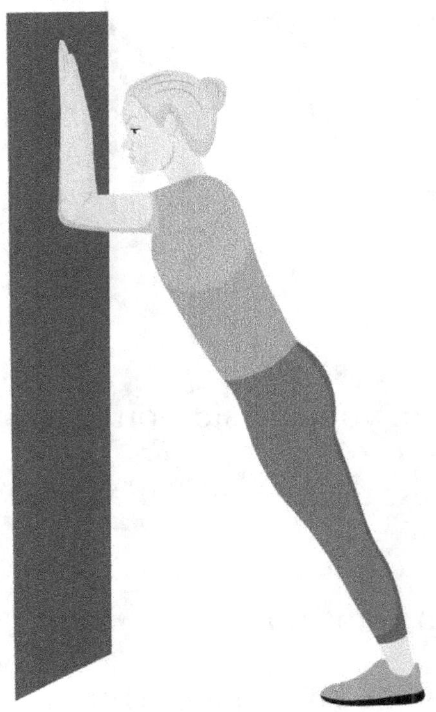

- Stand up and face the wall.

- Position your forearms against the wall while stepping back.

- Form a straight line from crown to heels.

- Tighten your core with every breath to prevent sagging or arching your back.

- Hold this position for 10 full breath counts.

Side Wall Lift

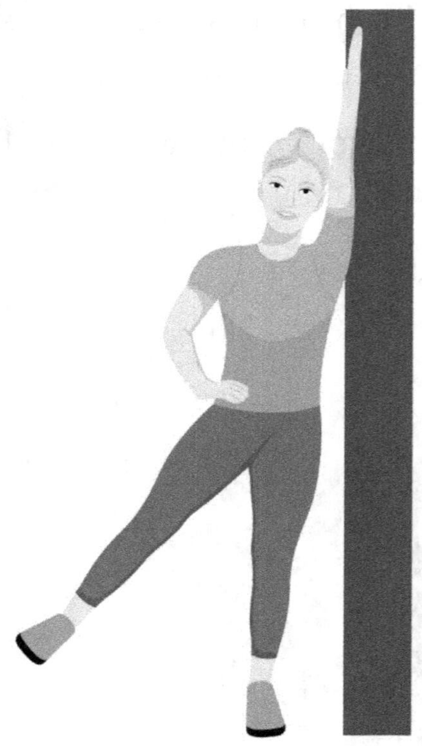

- Remain standing and align yourself side-on to the wall.

- Place your forearm closest to the wall flat against the wall, reaching up to the ceiling.

- Place your other hand on your hip.

- Now, lift your outer leg while ensuring the hips remain squared.

- Pulse your outer leg in small controlled movements for 10 pulses.

- Place your foot back on the floor.

- Turn around and align yourself side-on to the wall with the opposite side.

- Lift your outer leg while ensuring the hips remain squared.

- Pulse your outer leg in small controlled movements for 10 pulses.

- Place your foot back on the floor.

Dead Bug

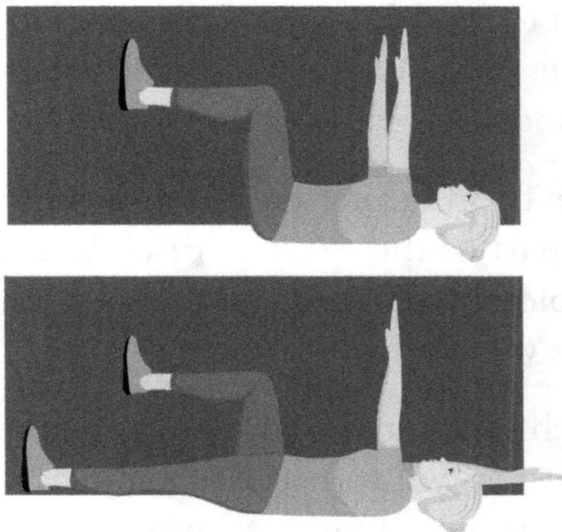

- Remain on the floor with legs bent at the knee and feet flat on the floor.

- Shift slightly away from the wall so only the tips of your fingers can touch the wall.

- Raise your arms out straight in front of you, reaching for the sky.

- Now, lower your left leg, straighten it, and lift your right leg, keeping your knee bent.

- While you are doing this, lower your left arm straight behind you, and bring your right arm to connect with your left knee.

- Shift and alternative between each side slowly, controlling your movements and your breath.

- Repeat 10 times.

This set of exercises may feel like quite a leap in the intensity of your workouts so take your time and make sure you're focusing on form rather than repetitions. If you're battling with these exercises, you may want to consider extending the workouts in weeks 1 and 2 or using the tips and tricks below to help modify your workout to suit your needs.

Adapting Exercises for Your Needs

This final section of week 3 focuses on personalizing and adapting your exercises. From fine-tuning each movement to modifying your exercises to meet your unique physical needs and goals, customizing your Wall Pilates drills ensures you can progress safely with maximum efficiency and strength-building.

Tailoring your exercises isn't something new and the different disciplines of Pilates encourage adaptation as a part of the exercise discipline. It's important to recognize that every one of us is completely different and that our range of motion, and strength on the mat (and against) the wall varies.

Personalizing your approach guarantees that your practice aligns perfectly with your body, enhancing your progress without risking injury. By listening attentively to your body and responding to its needs with modifications, you're creating a safe but progressive environment for yourself where you get stronger, more flexible, and continue to evolve in your Wall Pilates practices.

So what can you learn from this final section of Chapter 4 and how can you alter your routines to ensure optimal engagement?

Let's begin with the why—flexibility in modifying your workout is the key to your continued advancement. It provides you with the ability to face new fitness challenges while also considering the things that could possibly set you back physically. The ability to acknowledge your weaknesses is by no means a bad thing. In fact, it's an incredibly powerful way to analyze what needs work and tailoring to enhance your workouts and make them more enjoyable.

Now that you know why adaptation is important, let's take a look at how you can adapt your workouts.

1. **Use props for support:** Props like pillows, yoga blocks, or a small stability ball can provide you with both additional support and increased intensity of your workout, depending on how you interact with these tools. For example, laying a pillow behind your lower back can be used to offer extra comfort for some exercises or provide elevation for more intense workouts with other movements.

2. **Adjust your range of motion:** Modifying your range of motion accommodates any current limitations you may have while still strengthening your muscles. By gradually increasing or decreasing the range of motion of each of your movements, you can still progress in your workout intensity without the added worry of injuring yourself.

3. **Choose appropriate exercises:** If you already have a rock-solid core but your legs are weak, it's important that you place focus on balancing out your body. Opt for exercises that can be performed comfortably for stronger areas of your body and progress in intensity for areas that may be weaker.

4. **Slow and controlled movements matter:** prioritize slow and controlled movements over trying to reach the required repetition count. Rushing through exercises can put you at risk of hurting yourself and can set you back when it comes to your fitness journey.

5. **Listen to your body:** Always listen to your body and be mindful of any discomfort, pain, or dizziness. If a particular movement causes you to feel discomfort outside of the normal parameters of any healthy exercise, readjust, use additional modifications, or skip the exercise if absolutely necessary.

6. **Seated or lying positions:** Standing or weight-bearing exercises are challenging for some people and that is absolutely fine. If you're finding that you haven't quite progressed to standing poses, mix and match your workouts so that you are only participating in seated or lying positions.

7. **Consult with a professional:** If after working out and readjusting persistently you're still experiencing discomfort, you may want to consider consulting with a qualified Pilates instructor. They may be able to provide you with personalized advice based on your individual needs and limitations.

As you move through week 3, remember to honor your body, focus on your breath, and celebrate your progress. Some of us take longer than others to reclaim our fitness and strength but celebrating small wins will keep you motivated to continue improving. Before you know it, you'll be moving on to week 4 and more complex Wall Pilates workouts.

Chapter Five

Week 4: Advanced Techniques and Sequences

In this final week of Wall Pilates exercises, you'll begin to incorporate complex movements, introduce additional elements, like resistance bands and weights, and test your balance. Fair warning, the movements in this chapter are pretty complex and dynamic, so if you feel like you need to spend more time honing your techniques and building your strength, please feel free to do so. You'll notice this chapter is not labeled with a week number and that is because you will need decent strength, flexibility, and balance to take on these movements.

Having said that, there's no real harm in trying them out if you're doing so carefully and you're not putting yourself at risk of injury. Each of the movements in the workouts below is progressive. This means they will slowly increase in intensity, testing your limits, and ensuring you gain dynamic control over your body.

Make sure that you are setting aside adequate down and rest time between these workouts—I would suggest one full advanced workout per week to begin with, opting for less strenuous stretches, flexibility, balance, and beginner or intermediate workouts in between.

An Introduction to Advanced Leg Wall Pilates Techniques

For these exercises, you will need a small ball or firm pillow. To begin with, do not include additional weight as some of these exercises are incredibly taxing on the body. Once you are stronger, feel free to begin adding weight in the form of dumbbells or resistance in the form of a resistance band.

If this is your first time trying out the advanced exercises listed below, make sure that you are doing so safely and ask that someone be present in case of a fall. If no one is available, keep your phone on hand so that you can call someone in the case of an emergency.

Wall Sits

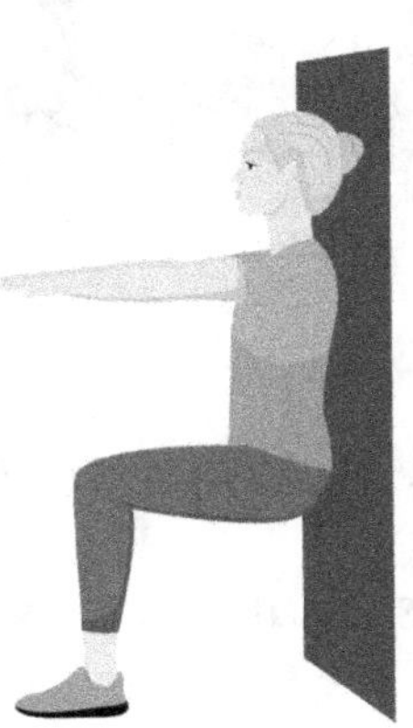

- Stand with your back against the wall.

- Take a good step forward to place about one and a half feet distance between your feet and the wall.

- Lift your arms straight out in front of your chest, palms facing the floor—for additional support, you can place your hands on your thighs, palms facing down.

- Inhale slowly and as you exhale, begin sliding your spine down the wall.

- Once you're in a sitting position, or where your muscles can comfortably hold you up, pause.

- Try to hold this position for 10 full breath counts but release and stand up if your muscles begin shaking or you feel unsteady.

Wall Clock Lunges

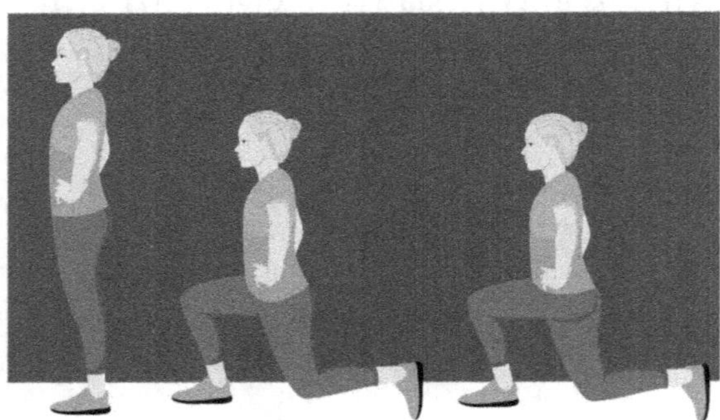

- Remain standing in your Wall Squat position.

- Place your hands on your hips, make sure your shoulders are relaxed, and your spine is straight.

- With your right leg, take a step to the right, bending your right knee as far as it will go—your left foot should be against the wall and your knee should be slightly bent.

- Return to your standing position.

- Take a step forward with your right leg this time, bending your right knee into a lunge position—your left foot should be against the wall and your knee slightly bent.

- Return to your standing position.

- Take a step to the left with your left leg this time, bending your left knee as far as it will go—your right foot should be against the wall and your knee should be slightly bent.

- Return to your standing position.

- Take a step forward with your left leg time, bending your left knee into a lunge position—your right foot should be against the wall and your knee slightly bent.

- Repeat this movement, alternating between legs for 5 full repetitions per leg, 10 in total.

One-Legged Wall Squat Hold

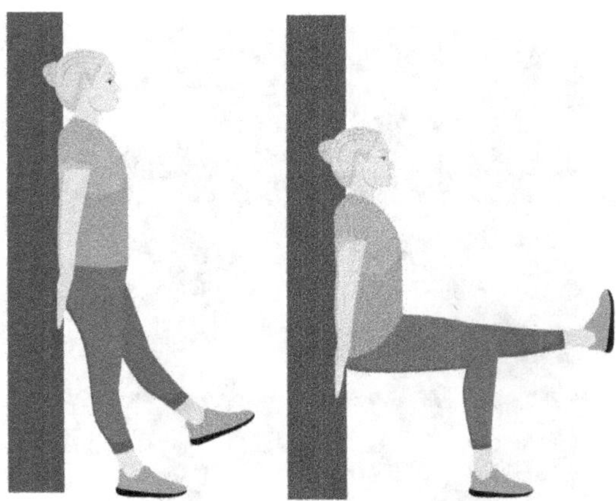

- Remain in your Wall Squat position, feet comfortably away from the wall.

- Place your arms at your side comfortably.

- Lift one leg off the floor and hold the position.

- If you're strong enough, begin to slide your back down the wall into a one-legged square position.

- Make sure your movement is controlled and comfortable.

- Hold the position for 5 breath counts.

- Return to your standing position.

- Now, repeat this movement with the other leg holding your weight.

- Hold the position for 5 breath counts.

Wall Stand & Squeeze

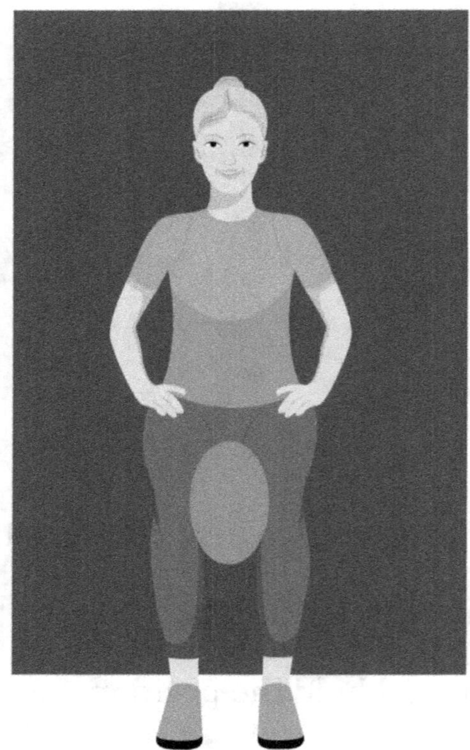

- Remain in your Wall Squat position.

- Pick up your pillow or ball and place it between your thighs, gripping it lightly with your knees.

- Place your hands on your thighs for support.

- Inhale and as you do, slowly lower your back down the wall.

- Do not enter into a full Wall Squat position. Rather have your knees slightly bent and be standing in a comfortable mini-squat position.

- Now, begin squeezing the ball/pillow.

- Squeeze with each inhale and release with each exhale being sure not to drop the ball/pillow.

- Aim to repeat for 10 full breath counts.

Wall-Supported Mountain Climbers

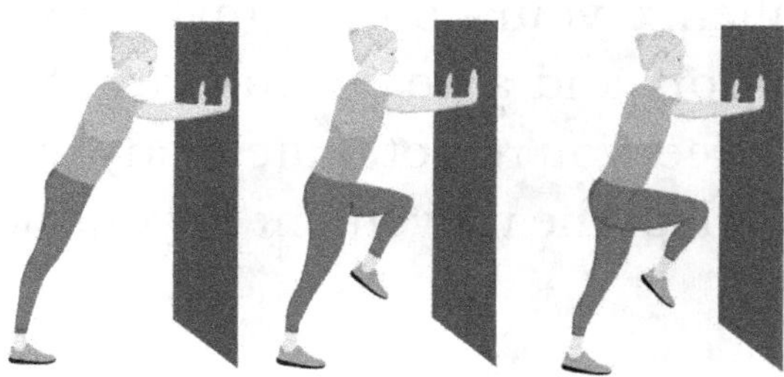

- Turn and face the wall, maintaining about one and a half feet between your feet and the wall, or more if you need it.

- Lean forward with slightly bent elbows, placing your palms flat on the wall in front of your palms facing up.

- Engage your core and inhale.

- Now, lift your right knee up toward your elbow, pausing for about half a breath count before placing it back on the floor.

- Do the same with your left knee in overly exaggerated marching movements.

- Alternate between legs for 10 full movements, 5 per leg.

Dynamic Sequences for Core Strength

Dynamic workouts are designed to elevate the intensity of a workout while improving the flow between each exercise. In this way, your Wall Pilates workout will begin to become a sequence of movements that works one set of muscles after the next. The purpose of dynamic workouts is to increase muscle endurance.

This set of dynamic workouts is specifically designed for your core and targets the different abdominal muscles as well as your back muscles to help support your core. Each routine has been designed to build stamina and improve the fluidity of your movements but is quite intense. Because of this, I encourage you to take the time to work on your form rather than repetitions. By spending more time on your form, you can increase the repetitions of each exercise in your own time and as your muscles adjust to the new intensity of your workouts.

Advanced Core Workout

These movements will challenge your body so make sure you are completing each exercise with the right support and a person nearby if possible. Your safety is of utmost importance so if you feel you're not quite ready to progress, replace a specific movement with another, or adapt the movement to your needs.

Elevated Wall Plank

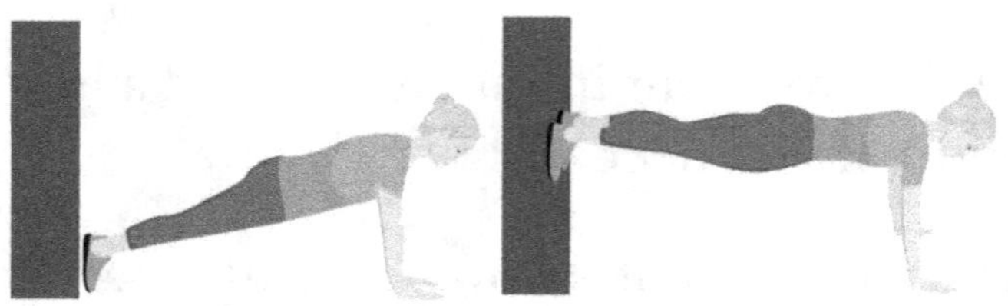

- Lie on your belly on the floor, feet flat against the wall.

- Place the palms of your hands on the floor just below your shoulders and as close to your body as possible.

- Inhale and lift your body off the floor using your arms.

- Now, begin to slide your feet up the wall with the aim of keeping your spine straight and in line with your shoulders.

- Hold this plank position for 10 full breath counts.

- **Note: This is a very advanced movement. If you cannot lift your feet up the wall, opt to keep them planted on the ground against the wall while keeping your body elevated with your arms.**

Pike-Up

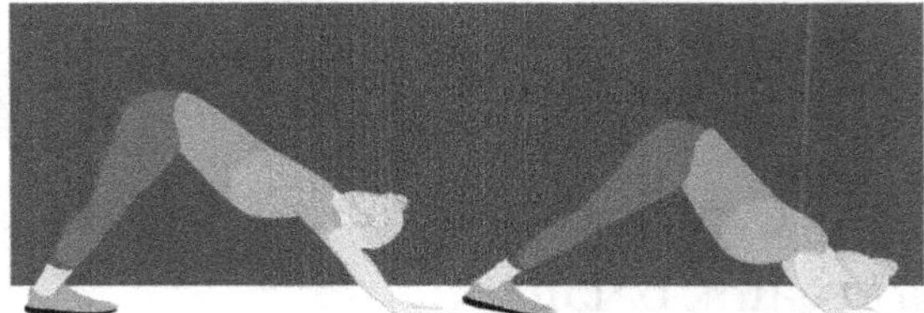

- Remain in your Wall Plank position.

- Place your hands on the floor with the palms of your hands next to your head at ear height.

- With your feet pressed against the wall, slowly lift your upper body off the floor.

- Engage your core and make sure it is doing most of the work and not your arms.

- Aim to form a V with your body.

- Hold this position, core engaged for 10 full breath counts.

- To intensify this movement, lift one hand off the ground and then the other, alternating between breaths.

V-Sit Ups

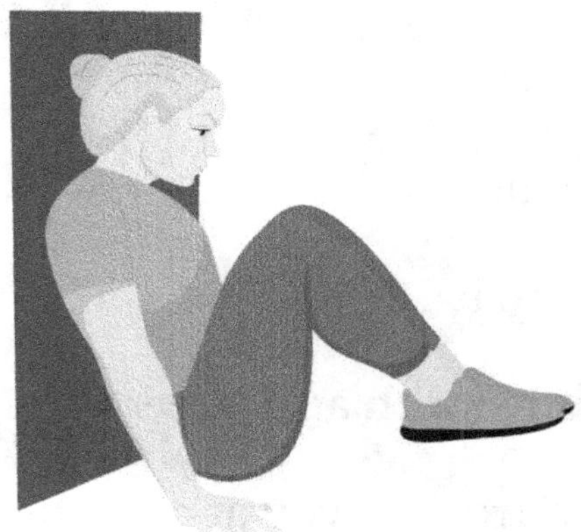

- Sit with your back against the wall, leaving a very small space between your behind and the wall.

- Place your hands on the ground next to you, palms on the floor.

- Place your legs straight out in front of you.

- Now, lift your feet and legs off the ground slightly, engaging your core and ensuring your body remains balanced.

- Slowly, bend your legs, bringing them to your abdomen until your body forms a v-shape.

- Hold for 2 breath counts and return your legs outstretched but do not place them on the floor.

- Repeat 10 full repetitions.

Wall Rotations

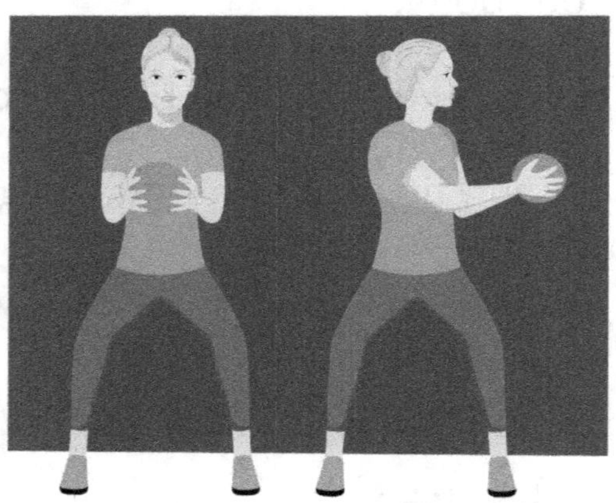

- Pick up your pillow or ball.

- Stand up and place your back against the wall.

- Open your legs about hip-width apart, feet facing forward.

- Hold your pillow/ball in front of you at chest height, elbows slightly bent.

- Slowly lower yourself into a comfortable mid-squat position.

- Inhale and as you exhale, twist your torso (not feet and legs) to the left.

- On your next inhale, return to the center.

- Next, exhale and twist your torso to the right.

- On your inhale, return to the center.

- Complete 10 full movements, 5 on each side.

Inverted Wall Crunch

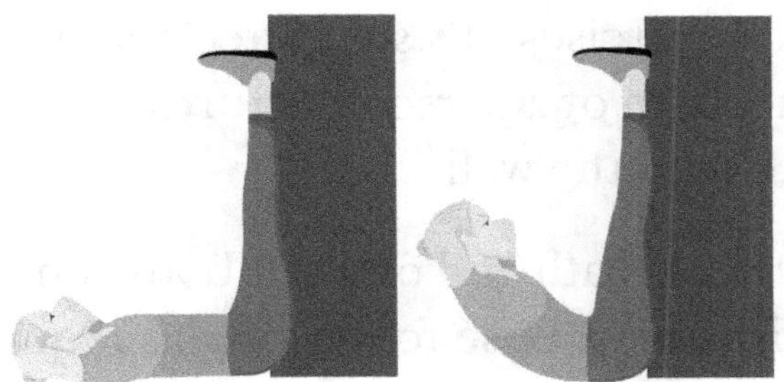

- Turn around but remain on the floor.

- Your behind needs to be flush against the wall and your legs straight up.

- Open your legs slightly so they form a V.

- Place your hands on your abdomen or on the floor for extra support.

- Inhale and as you exhale, lift your body off the floor, rolling your abdominal muscles.

- Aim to touch the wall and hold for your full exhale before returning to the floor.

- Complete 10 repetitions.

As mentioned before, these movements are quite intense and are designed to really target your abdominal muscles. Make sure you're not aiming for repetitions but for form and safety. Over time, you can build up the number of manageable repetitions for each of these movements.

Challenging Balancing Positions

Congratulations on making it through to the final set of exercises for your Wall Pilates workout routines. Did you know that 90% of people never complete what they have started, so you've done incredibly well?

This challenge is designed to elevate your balance positions. The complexity and flow of each of these movements not only cultivate stability but also enhance mental dexterity and control.

For these advanced balance exercises, it's suggested that you have an additional layer of balance protection in the form of a person or sturdy furniture nearby that allows for dual balance and resistance with the wall.

You will need to focus on your breath and on your body, finding your center of balance and concentrating on holding your pose for as long as required.

Advanced Balance Workout

Always make sure you're completing these exercises with safety at the forefront of your mind. Ensure you have your mobile phone or someone nearby who can assist while perfecting these poses.

Advanced Tree Pose

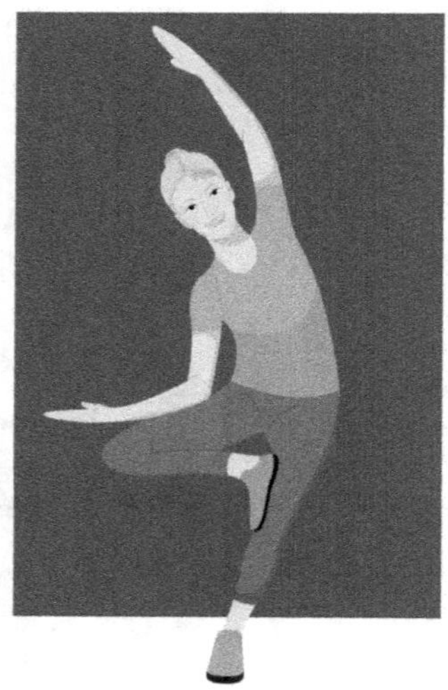

- Stand side-on with the wall, your hip should touch the wall when extended.

- Lift the arm closest to the wall above your head, placing your palm on the wall for initial balance.

- Lift your outer leg (the one furthest from the wall), bending it at the knee.

- Rest your foot on the inner thigh of your straight leg.

- Lift the arm furthest from the out, using it to balance.

- Now, slowly bend at the waist, resting your elbow on your bent leg.

- Your wall side should now be touching at the hip and make no contact with the wall other than this.

- Hold for 5 full breath counts.

- Shift sides, and complete the movement with the other side of your body.

Beside Handstand

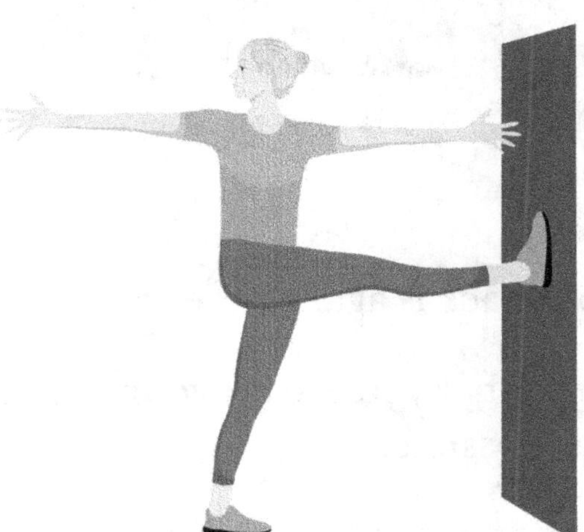

- Remain standing but turn and face the wall.

- With a sturdy piece of furniture, or someone to help you, lift your right leg off the floor and place it straight in front of you, your foot flat on the wall and toes pointing up.

- Inhale and as you exhale, lift your arms out to your sides.

- Straighten your arms and fingers and gently twist your torso in the direction of your lifted leg.

- Hold for 5 full breath counts.

- Carefully return to your standing position.

- Rebalance yourself and repeat with your left leg.

Pistol Squat and Hold

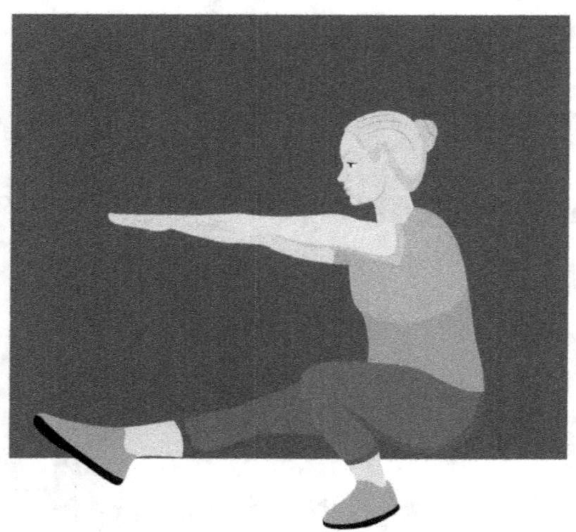

- Turn around so that your back is against the wall.

- Squat all the way down so that you are on your haunches, try to keep your feet as close to the ground as possible.

- Inhale and raise your hands out in front of you at chest height, arms straight.

- Make sure you are balanced and lift your left leg off the floor, aiming to straighten it out in front of you.

- Hold this position for 5 full breath counts.

- Return to your haunched starting position and rebalance yourself.

- When you are ready, lift your right leg off the floor, aiming to straighten it out in front of you.

- Hold this position for 5 full breath counts.

Floating Table

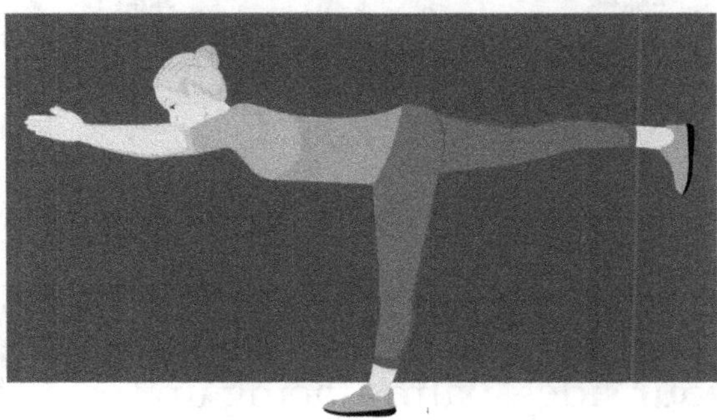

- Stand with your back to the wall.

- Take a large step forward, planting your feet on the ground and your toes facing forward.

- Inhale and lift your right leg, extending it backward to rest on the wall.

- As you exhale, lean forward, bending at the hips.

- Keep your spine straight and your arms straight out in front of you.

- Hold the position for 5 full breath counts.

- Return to a standing position, carefully.

- Rebalance yourself.

- Repeat the process with your left leg lifted and your right leg supporting your weight.

- Hold the position for 5 full breath counts.

Corpse Pose With Wall Resistance

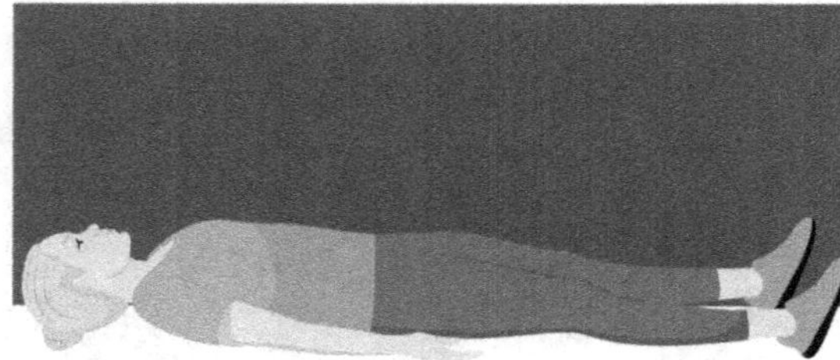

- Lay on the floor with your feet against the wall, legs straight and slightly open.

- Place your arms at your sides, palms facing up toward the ceiling.

- Flatten your spine against the floor.

- Inhale deeply and as you do, squeeze your core, drawing your belly downward toward your spine and filling your lungs with air.

- As you exhale, release your abdominal muscles, using them to push all of the air out of your lungs.

- Inhale once more, repeating this motion for 10 full breaths.

- Remain on the floor for a few seconds after this final pose.

- Slowly rise to your feet, opting to sit first and then stand so that you don't get dizzy.

Remember, these poses are advanced and it will take time to master them. Once you have, you can focus on moving seamlessly through each movement. Don't rush and remain safe at all times.

Creating Your Ongoing Practice Routine

As you conclude this final week of structured workouts, you may be wondering, *"How do I create an ongoing practice with the exercises I've learned?"*

Creating an ongoing practice routine is important as it helps solidify your new habits and ensure you are continually building upon your strength, balance, and flexibility.

This final chapter not only provides you with practical advice on maintaining your sessions but also supplies you with a suggested 28-day workout program. Outlining which days you can be used for which workouts, and ensuring you are able to have some rest and recovery in between, will provide you with a roadmap toward your continuous success.

Feel free to swap and change these workouts to fit with your schedule and don't forget to make use of your workout journal to record your progress as well as your workout for the day.

Tips and Tricks for Sustaining Your Workout Habit

Before reading the tips and tricks below, I'd like to highlight that your Wall Pilates workouts shouldn't feel like a chore. Try to incorporate your workouts at a specific time of the day when you know you won't be interrupted or have to rush. Have fun and work within your own goals, and always make sure that you are properly engaged and able to concentrate on what you're doing.

Set realistic goals: When setting your goals, be sure to be realistic, working within your current limitations. Choose to work on things that are meaningful to you like improving core strength, increasing flexibility, or alleviating back pain.

Start gradually: If you're new to Pilates or haven't exercised for a while, begin with less advanced exercises. Gradually introduce more challenging movements only when you are strong enough to and when you're confident with your abilities.

Establish a consistent schedule: It's normal to have ups and downs but consistency is key to success. With realistic goals and a sustainable schedule, you should be able to complete at least three workouts a week to ensure you're continually improving in strength, flexibility, and balance.

Shorter sessions can be effective too: With Wall Pilates, longer sessions are not necessarily more effective. Remember, these exercises are designed to really challenge your muscles so it's not necessary to overdo things.

Warm-up and cool down: Always warm up and cool down after and before a workout. Preparing your body for what is to come and allowing your muscles to cool down after an intense workout will minimize the risk of injury and reduce any muscle stiffness post-workout.

Stay hydrated and well-nourished: One of the biggest mistakes women make when it comes to a new fitness routine is neglecting nutrition. Make use of our upcoming free gift and make sure you're eating nourishing foods as well as hydrating well.

Always keep in mind that sustainability is about creating a routine that works for you and that you can maintain over time. Be consistent, enjoy your workouts, and nourish yourself well and you'll improve in leaps and bounds in no time.

Sample Workout Routine

The plan below is designed using the exercises contained in each of the previous chapters. Feel free to shift things around and remember to adhere to your rest days.

Week 1: Foundation Building

Day 1:

- Wall Press
- Wall Slide
- Wall Squats
- Rest

Day 2:

- Standing Wall Push
- Wall Cat Stretch
- Wall Sit-Ups

Day 3: **Rest**

Day 4:

- Wall Leg Pull-In
- Wall Crunches
- Wall Bridge

Day 5:

- Wall Plank

- Wall Arm Slide

- Wall Calf Stretch

Day 6: **Rest**

Day 7:

- Wall Chest Opener

- Wall Hamstring Stretch

- Wall Butterfly Stretch

Week 2: Progression and Challenge

Day 8:

- Wall-Supported Leg Pulls

- Wall Stand and Squeeze

- Wall-Mounted Tree Pose

Day 9:

- Wall Supported Warrior III

- Wall Angels

- One-Legged Wall Squat Hold

Day 10: **Rest**

Day 11:

- Standing Oblique With Breath

- Wall Posture Check

- Wall Pelvic Tilt

Day 12:

- Leg Ups With Breath

- Hip Opening Core Crunch

- Breath Pulse Squats

Day 13: **Rest**

- Wall Scapula Slide

- Wall Head Retraction

- Wall Stand and Reach

Day 14:

- Pelvic Curl Against the Wall

- Wall-Supported Knee Rolls

- Wall Supported Warrior III

Week 3: Intermediate Intensity

Day 15:

- Wall Child's Pose

- Wall Spine Straightener

- Wall Push-Offs

Day 16: **Rest**

Day 17:

- Wall Figure of Four

- Wall Scissors

- Leg Circles

Day 18:

- Wall-Supported Cobra Pose

- Chest and Shoulder Mobility Stretch

- Controlled Leg Extensions

Day 19: **Rest**

Day 20:

- Wall Sits

- Wall Clock Lunges

- One-Legged Wall Squat Hold

Day 21:

- Wall Bridge March

- Intermediate Wall Plank

- Side Wall Lift

Week 4: Advanced Challenges

Day 22:

- Wall Stand & Squeeze

- Wall Supported Mountain Climbers

- Dead Bug

Day 23: **Rest**

Day 24:

- V-Sit Ups

- Wall Rotations

- Elevated Wall Plank

Day 25:

- Inverted Wall Crunch

- Advanced Tree Pose

- Pike-Up

Day 26: **Rest**

Day 27:

- Floating Table

- Corpse Pose With Wall Resistance

- Beside Handstand

Day 28:

- Pistol Squat and Hold

- Wall Stand & Squeeze

- Wall Supported Mountain Climbers

You can adjust the intensity and repetitions based on your fitness, strength, and balance levels. Once you've progressed, feel free to add one exercise to every day, increasing the duration of each of your workouts.

Chapter Six

Addressing Female Aging with Wall Pilates

With our workouts now learned, it's important that we go into deeper depth when it comes to how Wall Pilates benefits us throughout our natural female aging processes. As we grow older, the fluctuations and changes in our hormone levels adjust our bone density and muscle mass and as a result, our strength, flexibility, and ability to avoid injury.

For us to properly manage the complex physiological changes happening in our bodies, we need to take control of not only our physical health in the form of diet and exercise but also our hormonal health.

I am a huge proponent of knowing all of the reasons why we need to institute change. Knowing the why provides us with the sustained motivation we need to overcome the mental hurdles we face on a daily basis as well as ensures we don't fall back into habits that are not great for our mental and physical health.

Added to this, when we understand why we are incorporating changes to our lifestyles, we can begin to become more empathetic with our personal journeys, choosing to uplift ourselves and understand that many of the limitations we're facing are not outside of our control.

Aging, when we embrace it and work to remain fit and healthy, is a privilege many before us haven't been afforded. What we need to understand is that it's about balance—not just of our perceptions of what someone over 50 should look or act like, but also the goals we set for ourselves as we age.

Understanding Female Aging and Physical Exercise

Women's bodies undergo distinctive changes as their hormones shift. As mentioned before, the primary change we experience from decreasing estrogen revolves around bone density and muscle mass. Having said that, we need to understand that estrogen is also absolutely critical to other systems and organs in our bodies. Estrogen affects the urinary tract and our ability to maintain bladder control, pelvic health, our skin, hair, the mucous membranes in our bodies, and even our ability to think clearly.

As our reproductive years draw to a close, estrogen slowly declines, plummeting through menopause. Women who have transitioned through the "change of life" may decide to take estrogen or progesterone/estrogen combined therapy to help combat issues like heart and degenerative neural diseases.

Now, I'm not saying that there isn't a place for modern medicine, because there is, but often hormone therapy treatments are pushed when women can adequately manage their hormonal health with natural alternatives to medicine. You see, after menopause, estrogen is produced by the adrenal glands and fatty tissues within our bodies. It's vitally important that estrogen remains balanced within the body because too little of the hormone signals trouble in the form of osteoporosis, heart disease, and coronary disease. Too much estrogen raises our risk of certain types of cancer and risk of stroke.

In postmenopausal women, physical exercise reduces the amount of estrogen that is free-flowing in the blood, balancing natural hormone levels within the body, and improves the symptoms associated with menopause.

Osteoporosis and Muscle Degradation After 50

Osteoporosis can dramatically impact our quality of life and aside from Western medicine treatments, prevention is better than cure. Having said that, a balanced diet rich in calcium and vitamin D as well as regular, moderate physical exercise is one of the most effective ways to combat osteoporosis.

Osteoporosis is characterized by low bone mineral density and the deterioration of bone tissue. Once osteoporosis has taken its grip, the risk of fractures, especially of the hip, spine, and wrist becomes a reality. There is some debate as to what the best form of exercise is to combat and reverse the effects of osteoporosis, but the general consensus is that controlled movement workouts that incorporate resistance are best.

The reason for this is that as bones are placed under moderate stress, new bone tissue begins to form, reinforcing the sites that were once weakened. Exercise is not a quick fix to osteoporosis though, and it takes consistency, a good diet, and gradual increases in intensity for us to safeguard against continued degradation.

The chapter that follows this one deals more specifically with nutrition and osteoporosis, but what is important to know right now is that your daily Wall Pilates workouts are helping your body regenerate. Brittle, calcium-deficient bones are being replaced with healthy tissue, and you are gaining strength, whether you're aware of it or not.

Muscle degradation, also known as sarcopenia, occurs for a number of reasons including illness, a sedentary lifestyle, and a lack of confidence in our ability to increase the intensity of our workouts. Diet and age-related changes in hormone levels and metabolism also factor into how quickly our muscles will degrade.

When we increase the intensity and resistance of our workouts, micro-tears occur within the muscle fibers of our bodies. These tears stimulate the body to begin repairing our muscles by adding protein and water. This in turn builds the size and strength of the muscle.

Exercises that are compound in their nature, like Wall Pilates, use multiple muscles, working out not just large groups of muscles but also the fine muscles that are required for balance and coordination.

Both exercise and diet are incredibly important to muscle health—and no, I'm not talking about eating like a rabbit either. For muscles to grow and maintain adequate strength, we need a diet that is rich, varied and contains adequate protein (but more on that a bit later).

The huge plus about Wall Pilates as a primary form of exercise as we age is that it provides not just the resistance we need but also the stability required to protect against falls. It promotes balance and coordination, and by default reduces the risk of a fall. What we need to do is build our confidence in our body's ability to perform the movements, building ourselves up gradually until gains are felt. Remember, the low-impact nature of Wall Pilates exercises provides you with a safe, accessible, and beneficial workout that you can tailor-make for yourself.

Pilates for Hormonal Balance and Menopause Management

Menopause signals a turbulent time in many of our lives. It's not just our physical state but our emotional, mental, and psychological states as we tussle with the idea that we're getting older.

On a physical level, some of us experience disturbed sleep, wild fluctuations in our emotions, hot flashes, headaches, and intense muscle pain, while others may get away with relatively mild symptoms. The severity of our symptoms, however, are not an indication of what is happening in our bodies and we need to understand what is happening inside us so that we can manage not only the symptoms that may be experienced but also any potential damage happening.

Physical activity is vital to hormone management and the precarious balancing act we unwittingly enter into after the age of 50. By remaining active we can minimize the effects of reducing hormone levels, and increase key neurochemicals essential for mental well-being and the production of Estrone (E1), the milder form of estrogen our bodies produce after menopause.

Several studies suggest that regular, consistent physical exercise may have more of an effect on hormone balance than medication alone, here are some examples.

- Resistance exercise that works the muscles produces testosterone, a hormone that boosts physical energy and sex drive.

- Low and moderate-intensity workouts release endorphins, our feel-good neurochemical that balances well-being and encourages our body to produce other hormones.

- Exercise regulates cortisol production, an essential secondary hormone responsible for Estrone production.

- Consistent muscle-tiring workouts promote the healthy release of serotonin and melatonin, the hormones responsible for good-quality sleep.

- The addition of muscles helps burn calories in the body more effectively, fighting issues like insulin resistance, diabetes, and cardiovascular disease.

- Finally, resistance-type exercise promotes the release of human growth hormone which is critical for bone and muscle health.

The advantages of Wall Pilates as a way to manage hormonal imbalances as we age are unlimited, but once again, it's important to note that consistency and diet are key to effective change.

Mindfulness, Wall Pilates, and Mental Well-Being

One of the biggest knocks I took when I turned 50 was to my mental health. My kids had all left home and some had started families of their own after so many years in the corporate world, I found myself at home, bored, and often quite lost at what to do with this phase of my life.

I had read about mindfulness and breathwork practices but it wasn't something I wanted to do as a standalone practice. I think being caught up in my own thoughts didn't help and sitting in quiet contemplation only led to racing thoughts.

One of the biggest perks I found after starting with my Wall Pilates routine was that my mind calmed. The stress and anxiety that plagued me subsided without much conscious effort or mental work and I found it so interesting that I began to dive into the research.

What I found out is that Wall Pilates, with its smooth, controlled movements and focus on breathing had begun calming both my mind and body, allowing me to relax while strengthening my muscles, stretching away tension, and helping to soothe my anxiety.

The reason for this is that Wall Pilates practices are a form of mindfulness movement that boosts mood by releasing feel-good endorphins along with dopamine and serotonin. The best part about Wall Pilates workouts is that the effect of your workout lasts for hours and not just while you're exercising and over time, the consistent base-level elevation of these hormones improves mild to moderate depression and anxiety.

Wall Pilates also aids in facilitating good quality sleep by improving circulation and releasing the relaxing neurotransmitters required for healing, restorative sleep. This, in turn, lifts brain fog, improves cognitive function, and allows us to remain focused when it's needed the most.

Including Wall Pilates in your daily routines is a great way to engage your mind as well as your body. The combination of physical challenge, mental focus, and improved self-confidence allows you to build a holistic outlook on your overall well-being and health.

What is critical to understand, though, is that as with any holistic, more natural approach to health, it takes time and consistent effort to undo years of not knowing how to care for your aging body properly. Having the knowledge provides you with all of the reasons you should place your time, effort, and focus on building a healthy, strong, body so that you can age with grace, comfort, and pain-free.

Chapter Seven

Nutrition and Hydration for Optimal Results

As we venture into our 50s and beyond, we need to place more focus on our nutrition and hydration needs. The reason for this renewed focus is now different from our earlier years when a svelte figure and society's standards had us chasing impossible beauty standards.

Now, the emphasis is placed on overall health, well-being, hormonal balance, and fueling the new muscle and bones we are creating. This chapter will help unlock some of the most powerful secrets science has to offer when it comes to nutrition over the age of 50, allowing you to harness the power of properly nourishing your body.

The path to well-being and renewed strength begins with mindful eating and paying attention to the essential nutrients, vitamins, and minerals that form the cornerstone of healing and supporting our bodies. Nourishing our bodies with a well-balanced diet rich in whole foods, vibrant produce, lean proteins, and healthy fats ensures we are supporting health on a cellular level and working to ramp up our flailing metabolism.

Beyond the foods we will discuss in this chapter, and their roles, we'll discuss how to properly hydrate your body to improve joint flexibility, aid in muscle generation, and preserve cognitive function. Contrary to popular belief, you don't need to be downing gallons of water to meet your hydration criteria and many women over the age of 50 do more damage to their bodies overhydrating than under hydrating—but more on that later.

The Importance of Nutrition in Exercise and Aging

Proper nutrition plays an absolutely critical role in building muscle mass and maintaining the health of our muscles. I can't overstate this point, what you eat directly impacts the body's ability to strengthen itself, repair damage, and maintain muscle and bone mass. Because we're already fighting a bit of a losing battle when it comes to maintaining muscle mass, we need to ensure that we're fueling ourselves properly.

As women age their body's nutritional needs evolve, and this is particularly true when it comes to muscle health. Eating properly and nourishing our bodies not only provides the energy and sustenance needed to perform physical activities but also supplies us with the essential building blocks necessary to repair and grow muscles. That means that eating a diet that is balanced and includes a variety of nutrients is really for supporting muscle health, strength, and functionality.

Ironically, as we age, our bodies seem to crave less protein but this essential nutrient is incredibly important for muscle health. Protein is composed of amino acids, the fundamental building blocks of muscle tissue, and when we engage in physical activities, especially exercise routines like Wall Pilates, the demand for amino acids increases. The reason for this is that our body is stimulated to repair the micro tears that occur when we exercise. Added to this, proteins are essential for maintaining the body's muscle mass and strength while aging because of the inherent nature of muscle loss during the aging process.

We cannot, however, neglect our carbohydrate intake. Carbs are seen as big evils in the world of restrictive dieting but the reality is that they serve as a primary source of energy for our bodies during physical activities. Carbohydrates are stored as glycogen which provides us with the necessary energy for muscle contractions and movement.

While it is true that fat can also be converted to glucose, it cannot directly be converted to the glycogen needed to fuel a workout. Healthy fats need to undergo a process in the body to be converted to glucose first, a longer-burning fuel.

This means that these healthy fats, like Omega-3 fatty acids, are used for long-term recovery and energy while carbohydrates are used immediately while an action or movement is taking place.

With all of this in mind, it becomes more evident why we need to eat in a more balanced way to facilitate muscle repair, maintain muscle and organ health, and have enough immediate and sustained energy to perform daily workouts. Proper nutrition also ensures we are taking into account our overall overall well-being, reducing the risk of chronic conditions and promoting a healthy aging process.

What to Eat for Muscle and Bone Health

The good news is that we can eat for healthy bones and muscles. Saying we should eat a balanced and varied diet to support muscle development and maintenance is one thing, but actually knowing what to eat is completely different.

- **Proteins:** I know it's been drummed into you already but protein is important. Having said that, not all protein is made equal and you're going to need to select high-quality protein lean meats, poultry, fish, eggs, dairy products, legumes, and plant-based proteins, like soy and quinoa as your first choices.

- **Calcium and vitamin D:** These two fundamental minerals and vitamins are critical for maintaining healthy bones. A lack of calcium is the leading cause of bone fragility and a higher risk of fractures. Calcium can be sourced from whole-fat dairy products, leafy green vegetables, kale and broccoli, almonds, and fortified plant-based milk. Vitamin D is synthesized from being in the sun but can also be obtained from eating fatty fish, egg yolks, and certain fortified foods, like cereals, grains, and orange juice.

- **Magnesium, phosphorus, and potassium:** These essential minerals support bone density, strength, and a healthy pH balance. Foods in these three mineral groups include nuts, seeds, whole grains, leafy green vegetables, dairy products, lean meat, and legumes.

- **Omega-3 fatty acids:** Found in fatty fish, flaxseeds, and walnuts, this healthy fat aids in muscle recovery and in supporting bone density. Added to this, Omega-3 possesses anti-inflammatory properties to help keep pain and inflammation at bay.

Many of the foods in our bone and muscle strength section overlap which makes it easier to manage eating a varied diet. Making informed choices about what you're eating can help you achieve your health and fitness goals quicker and ensure that you're supporting your body as it transitions into a new phase of life.

Food and Hormone Health

Not many women know that food and nutrients can play a critical role in how well our hormones remain balanced after the age of 50. Hormone shifts and fluctuations can impact our physical and mental health, and by eating for our hormones, we can influence and manage the side effects associated with these fluctuations.

As we know, physical exercise, particularly resistance and muscle-tiring workouts like Wall Pilates plays a massive role in hormone management. With regular, consistent physical exercise you can minimize the effects of declining hormone levels, increase essential neurochemicals for mental well-being, and balance natural hormone levels within your body. But, diet is also a key player in managing hormone levels and overall health.

Age-related changes in hormone levels and metabolism when combined with factors like illness and a sedentary lifestyle, can influence the rate at which your muscles degrade. Proper nutrition, therefore, is vitally important for hormone balance. Of course, a balanced diet is important and if you're eating for muscle and bone strength, then chances are you're already well on your way to great hormonal health. For a more specific list of hormone-balancing foods, take a look below.

- **Cruciferous vegetables:** Broccoli, cauliflower, Brussels sprouts, and kale contain compounds that support estrogen metabolism and contribute to hormone balance.

- **Flaxseeds:** These little powerhouses are rich in lignans and have been studied for their potential to modulate estrogen levels and support hormonal balance.

- **Avocados:** Packed with monounsaturated fats, avocados support overall hormone production.

- **Berries:** Rich in antioxidants and fiber, berries like blueberries, strawberries, and raspberries support overall health.

- **Legumes:** Beans and lentils are sources of plant-based protein and nutrients that contribute to hormone balance, they're also great sources of fiber.

- **Turmeric:** Long used in herbal medicine, turmeric contains curcumin, a compound that has been studied for its potential to modulate estrogen.

- **Greek yogurt:** This natural yogurt is a source of probiotics and protein that are great for your gut health and metabolism as a whole.

- **Pomegranates:** Another antioxidant powerhouse, pomegranates have been studied for their potential to influence estrogen levels in the body.

- **Seaweed:** The ocean's iodine source, seaweed is rich in other nutrients too, and is known for its potential to support thyroid health and hormonal balance.

Incorporating these foods into a balanced diet provides you with a whole lot of different options that can help positively influence hormone levels and support overall hormonal health. While many of the foods listed above have been widely studied, it's important to note that individual responses can vary. It's not advisable to eat a diet that is overly hormone-rich—remember balance is key when it comes to nutrition and exercise.

Hydration Fundamentals for Over 50s

Staying hydrated is important for our overall health and well-being but for women over 50, it's particularly important. Proper hydration is essential for maintaining bodily functions, supporting vital organs, and ensuring our brains work optimally.

The issue with hydration in women is that generally speaking we come from two different schools of thought: The water is disgusting group and the "We love H20" group. Here's the thing about water, like diet and exercise, it's a balancing act—too much water isn't good for you, too little is asking for trouble, and drinking it too quickly can cause imbalances.

That's right! You can down a gallon of water and hope that's your fill for the day because chances are, that water is going to just pass right through you. Before we get into hydration fundamentals though, let's take a look at why proper hydration is important.

1. **Maintaining cognitive function:** Proper hydration is essential for supporting cognitive function, memory recall, and overall mental clarity.

2. **Supporting hormonal health:** Proper hydration helps regulate hormones and the management of any extra hormones you may have floating around your body.

3. **Bone and joint health:** Hydrating properly supports the lubrication of joints and

the maintenance of bone density.

4. **Digestive health:** Proper hydration supports digestive function, ensuring we are properly absorbing the nutrients we are eating.

Actionable Tips and Tricks to Ensure Hydration

- **Set reminders:** Let's face it, just because we're no longer working doesn't mean we're not still juggling a whole lot of balls. Setting reminders to drink water at regular intervals throughout the day can jog your memory and make sure you don't skip your water for the day.

- **Hydrating foods:** There are a lot of foods that have a high water content which can help you keep up with your hydration. These include watermelon, cucumbers, and oranges.

- **Carry a marked bottle:** Keeping a refillable water bottle on hand to help keep visual track of how much water you've had for the day.

- **Monitor urine color:** Dark or cloudy urine is not a good sign. Keep an eye on the color of your urine for a simple but effective indicator of how hydrated you are.

- **Drink herbal teas:** If you're not a big water drinker, herbal teas like chamomile or peppermint can provide you with the extra hydration you need.

- **Limit alcohol and caffeine:** The odd drink or cup of coffee is fine but caffeine and alcohol are very dehydrating. Keep an eye on your caffeine and alcohol consumption and up your water after drinking these two items.

- **Keep it varied:** Water is great for you but too much of it can throw electrolytes out of balance. Make sure to have a variety of liquids like coconut water, herbal infusions, and natural fruit juices so that you have a diverse selection of healthy fluids to drink.

Hydration is important, especially when incorporating activity and exercise into your life. Make sure you are prioritizing what you're drinking, and how much as part of your daily healthy body practices.

A Word On Anti-Inflammatory Foods for Joint Health

Proper nutrition can do wonders for those aches and pains that accompany aging. Inflammation is a natural response to damage or illness in our bodies but can sometimes run rampant if left unchecked. Certain foods are known for their anti-inflammatory properties and will help you keep your inflammation in check, adding an additional layer of protection to your joints.

- **Omega-3 fatty acids:** Coming in as a bone, muscle, hormone, and joint-healthy food, Omega-3s are a known powerhouse for their anti-inflammatory properties. Sources of Omega-3 fatty acids include fatty fish, flaxseeds, chia seeds, and walnuts.

- **Vitamin C:** An essential antioxidant and collagen synthesis vitamin, vitamin C contributes to the maintenance of healthy connective tissues and joints. Citrus fruits, strawberries, kiwi, and bell peppers are all excellent sources of vitamin C.

- **Collagen-rich foods:** There is some debate in the scientific community as to whether or not collagen can be consumed and used within the body but there's no harm in trying. Some sources of collagen-rich foods include bone broth and chicken skin.

- **Ginger:** This is another anti-inflammatory powerhouse known for its ability to reduce inflammation and support joint health.

- **Sulfur-containing foods:** Sulfur is essential for the production of naturally occurring collagen in the body. Sulfur foods include garlic, onions, and cruciferous vegetables, including broccoli and Brussels sprouts.

Other foods that are listed under hormone and bone and muscle health are also great for your joints and the synthesis of collagen in the body. Remember, water and being properly hydrated are just as important to healthy, flexible joints so make sure you are drinking enough liquids.

Free Gift

Still not sure how to incorporate these healthy foods into your diet? Scan the QR code below to gain access to your free copy of our exclusive recipe book. Here, you'll find a selection of foods and their accompanying recipes to help support a healthy, balanced diet. Each recipe has been carefully sourced, ensuring you are not only getting the nutrients you need but also that there are meals tailored to every budget.

Chapter Eight

Integrating Pilates Into Your Lifestyle

Getting older can mean we fill our time with more things we enjoy doing in a bid to fill the gap work once filled. Integrating Wall Pilates into our daily routines can help us to find a balance between the things that are healthy for us as well as the things we do to relax and have some much-deserved downtime.

The significant changes in our bodies and our lifestyles require us to adapt and change not just our approach to fitness but to our mental and emotional well-being. Wall Pilates offers us a more holistic approach to a sometimes difficult life transition.

With your recipes and meal plan now downloaded, your exercise routine provided, and shifting our attention to sustainably integrating Wall Pilates and the other practices we've learned into our daily lives. This chapter focuses less on your exercise and diet and more on what you can do to complement your Wall Pilates practice for a well-rounded and balanced life. From tips and tricks in complementing current routines to other healthy lifestyle changes you can make, and nurturing your mental health with a more mindful approach to life, your years after 50 can become a pivotal positive turning point for you.

Complementing Current Lifestyles

We'll begin by saying that just because you're incorporating a healthier approach to life doesn't mean you need to experience a massive upheaval. On the contrary, Wall Pilates, mindfulness, and great eating habits can be slowly integrated into your current lifestyle. Creating a sustainable exercise habit that allows you to still continue to enjoy your life affords you the opportunity to shift your current mindset that exercise has to be a chore and that dieting means starving yourself.

The first thing you're going to need to know about integrating Wall Pilates, or any other change for that matter, is that it's about becoming aware of old habits that aren't great for you. Spending three hours on the sofa binge-watching a series is counterproductive because it does nothing for your mental, physical, or spiritual health. Becoming aware of how you are spending your time means you can find the gaps in your current routines that could be used to improve your quality of life.

The next, and very important aspect of making any change in your life is to know why you're doing what you're doing in the first place. This involves setting realistic goals for yourself when it comes to a balanced way of life. Look at the different areas of your life and decide what you'd like to improve upon, set goals for each of these areas, and then break each of these goals down into much smaller milestones that can be achieved. You don't want to overwhelm yourself with new tasks and goals, so focus on one small change every day and before you know it, you'll begin to see and feel a big difference. Consistency over intensity is absolutely critical to effective and sustainable change.

One of the biggest benefits when it comes to Pilates as a discipline is that it's not just about a strong, svelte body. It's about mindfulness, breathwork, and precision in your movements. By embracing the principles of Wall Pilates in all areas of your life, you can begin to institute small positive changes while still remaining focused on the things you enjoy about your current lifestyle.

For people who prefer a more solitary practice, it can be really helpful to set up a dedicated space that is both practical and welcoming. Have your equipment on hand, replace towels after every workout, and stock up on some easy-to-grab snacks. Alternatively, if you're a more social person and you have the space, why not invite some friends over to make your Wall Pilates workouts a fun group activity?

Above everything else, remember to be kind and recognize that the changes you are making are a process. Recognize your progress rather than what you think you should be achieving, and nurture yourself with self-care practices that celebrate your victories, no matter how small you believe them to be.

Ready For a Bigger Challenge: Combining Wall Pilates with Other Activities

The beauty of Wall Pilates is that they're short, targeted, workouts that are incredibly effective. This means that you can opt to increase the intensity of your workout by adding more resistance and weight (refer to Chapter 10 for more details), or begin taking on other forms of exercise that compliment your Wall Pilates practices.

Below are some 50-plus-friendly physical activities that both complement your Wall Pilates workouts and help to keep you fit and healthy.

1. **Walking and hiking:** Consistently-paced walks twice a week are great for your cardiovascular health and can enhance your core strength and overall stability. Make sure that you are walking in a safe place with even ground and in a group. Keep your phone on hand and always remain hydrated and well-nourished.

2. **Swimming:** Pairing Wall Pilates is a smart and effective way to engage in low-impact, full-body workouts. While Pilates works to strengthen your core and improve posture, swimming adds a layer of resistance while still being easy on the joints.

3. **Yoga:** As your balance and flexibility improve, you may look for ways to deepen and enhance these aspects of your health. Yoga is a great Wall Pilates companion that aids in supporting posture alignment and mindful muscle engagement.

4. **Gardening:** Getting involved in outdoor gardening practices is a great way to test out your newfound balance and coordination skills and get the vitamin D your body needs for good, strong bones. Added to this, gardening deepens the shoulder, back, and arm muscles workouts you get when enjoying Wall Pilates.

5. **Dance and other mindful movements:** Dancing, Tai Chi, and even painting sessions require both coordination and thoughtful movement. Engaging in other forms of mindful movement can enhance your Wall Pilates workouts, strengthen your muscles, and keep your cognitive functioning in tip-top shape.

There is nothing wrong with adding other forms of exercise to your life, in fact, I encourage it! An effective fitness routine is one that supports your overall health and well-being. As long as you're consistent in your practices and make time for regular workouts you enjoy alongside Wall Pilates, your body will become stronger and healthier over time.

Mindfulness Outside of Pilates

Mindfulness may be based on ancient practices but it has fast become one of the most studied modern Western tools to promote well-being. All mindfulness is, is the ability to consciously shift your focus between internal and external stimuli without judgment.

Mindfulness can be developed through meditation, mindful movement practices like Wall Pilates, and learning to manage your emotions through self-care and non-judgmental acknowledgment of your feelings and emotions.

Neuroscience shows that mindfulness has a significant impact on improving cognitive function well into our 70s and the reason for this lies in our ability to remember information, orient ourselves spatially, and think in unconventional ways. Wall Pilates does all of that, teaching us different movements, allowing us to shift and orient ourselves to our environment, and using the wall and other sturdy pieces of furniture for additional leverage.

Aside from your Wall Pilates workouts, it is beneficial to add mindfulness to other areas of your life, paying attention to the things that are important, and choosing to actively engage in your environment as often as possible. Below are some other ways you can incorporate mindfulness. Some of these, like controlled breathing, will need to be consciously incorporated into your workouts, while others, like focusing your thoughts and movements happen more naturally.

- Control your breathing, choosing to focus on your conscious breath.

- Choosing to remain grounded in the here and now rather than living in the past or future.

- Managing your emotions by acknowledging and accepting them and then shifting your focus to something else.

- Paying attention to what you're doing and consciously engaging with your environment.

- Including mindfulness in smaller areas of your life, like food preparation, eating, bathing, and getting dressed.

- Setting aside time to stretch and feel the movements of your body.

- Learning to accept where you are in your life and understanding that the only influence we have over anything is the actions we take to improve our lives.

Mindfulness is a powerful, science-backed tool that you can use not just in your workout routines but in your day-to-day life. It helps to keep you grounded and over time, becomes a cornerstone to a more peaceful, joyous, and content life, regardless of the fact that we are aging.

Added to this, mindfulness provides us with the confidence we need to continue to grow, develop, and adapt to a new way of life as we age, and encourages us to embrace the newly unfolding chapters of our lives.

Staying Motivated and Positive

There are going to be times when your motivation wanes—maybe often in the beginning too. This is natural! Motivation is a temporary state that often fails us before self-discipline and habits form and it's important that we know how to reignite our motivation so that we can progress with our workouts and healthy lifestyle.

This final section of our chapter on creating sustainable Wall Pilates habits that we can integrate into our current lifestyles focuses on how we can create routines that will become habits that don't require us to continually motivate ourselves. Adopting a positive mindset and embracing the changes we have set for ourselves is the first step but here is how we can move forward using the power of habit-formation.

1. **Use your free gift to track your progress and set goals**: Constantly reassess your goals as you begin to progress and look at areas of your life that may require new and improved habits.

2. **Create a schedule and stick to it**: Treat your exercise, eating, and mindfulness time as an important appointment. Show up on time, be prepared, and prioritize it over anything else that may come up.

3. **Include friends and family**: Even if you're working out alone, it's important to share your successes with others. A sense of belonging and having a group of people who support your fitness journey will keep you both motivated and accountable.

4. **Focus on the benefits**: When you find your motivation waning, remind yourself of all of the positive benefits of your workout routines and your healthy diet. Improved energy, better sleep, and improved mood are all good ways to become motivated.

5. **Mix it up**: Just because you have a routine set out for you doesn't mean you need to stick to it. As long as you're incorporating a Wall Pilates workout on your given days, you're progressing.

Finally, remember why you started this journey. Adopting Wall Pilates as part of a clearly defined goal for better health and well-being. Remain focused on whatever your personal reason for buying this book and choosing to become active after the age of 50. And, most importantly, be consistent in your practices—it takes on average only two months for a new habit to form.

Chapter Nine

Troubleshooting Common Wall Pilates Issues

As you venture deeper into our Wall Pilates practice, it's normal to encounter some hiccups or issues along the way. Your body is an intricate system, so it makes sense that not everything will go smoothly right off the bat. The key is addressing these issues compassionately and making adjustments to continue safely progressing. This introduction will deal with some of the more common issues you can expect to face when beginning with Wall Pilates, but the chapter as a whole will provide you with effective tips that can be used to overcome more unexpected or bigger obstacles.

Some of the more common issues you can expect to face is shoulder or neck strain when doing exercises that involve extended arms or overhead movements. This discomfort often stems from a lack of mobility in the upper back or long-held tension in the shoulders. The solution? Always warm up with shoulder rolls and rotations to lubricate the joints. Move slowly into overhead reaches, back off if there's pinching, and use a chair or block to decrease the range of motion until your upper back gets stronger. Proper alignment also helps take unwanted stress off the neck, so focus on stacking your joints and drawing the shoulders down.

Another hiccup is lower back pain during core exercises. The cause typically lies in weak abdominal muscles that force the back to overwork and that's why Wall Pilates is great—because it targets the very muscles that cause you to suffer from lower back pain in the first place. Aside from including core workouts two to three times a week, belly breathing and mindful breath techniques will help to strengthen your core and help you become more in tune with your body so that you can engage your core when necessary.

Finally, another common issue is hand, wrist, or elbow discomfort. Joint prep is key, as is going easy on any movements with straight arms like Side Planks. Bend elbows, and lower to forearms, or take breaks to alleviate pain. Strengthening the arms and releasing tension through self-massage helps long-term.

Ultimately, it's up to you to listen to your body and adjust as needed. Be compassionate with yourself, especially if you need to take a few extra sessions to build capacity before progressing. Wall Pilates isn't a sprint. It's a marathon where you get to experience the joy that comes from moving with purpose. Try not to become frustrated by not achieving an advanced posture immediately. Keep breathing, focus on good form, and trust that consistency will carry you through the occasional hiccups on your Pilates journey.

Overcoming Plateaus in Wall Pilates

Hitting a plateau while doing your Wall Pilates routine is common and can be frustrating. You feel like you've stopped making progress or certain moves that used to challenge you now seem too easy. Plateaus are a normal occurrence and it's not something to be particularly concerned about unless you find that you have been doing your workouts consistently for months and feeling no progress whatsoever. In the case of no progress, it's important to consult with a healthcare professional who can help you find out what underlying health issues may be stalling progress.

Aside from real medical issues, taking leaps forward and backward happens and you can overcome plateaus by trying the tips below.

1. **Analyze your technique:** Focus on perfecting your technique and form in the Wall Pilates moves you currently do. Are you maintaining proper alignment, stacking joints, and engaging the right muscles? Mastering the small details will help you advance to more difficult variations even if you remain at the same overall exercise. For example, work on performing a controlled Roll Down with perfect posture before attempting it with small weights.

2. **Increase resistance:** Add resistance bands or small hand weights to basic moves to make them more challenging without having to progress to an advanced exercise. This forces your body to work harder while still doing familiar movements. Start with 1-3 lb weights and light resistance bands, increasing resistance over time—we'll discuss this in-depth in the next chapter.

3. **Slow the pace:** Performing Wall Pilates exercises at a slower, more controlled pace increases time under tension for your muscles and up the difficulty. Use a 3 count for the lowering phase and a 5 count for the lifting phase. You'll feel the burn even with beginner moves when you focus on slowly controlled movement.

4. **Cross-train with some form of cardiovascular exercise:** If you feel like your Wall Pilates workout isn't working up a sweat, it may be time to add some cardio training to the mix. Swimming, walking, hiking, and even dancing can help raise your heart rate and provide that little bit of extra intensity you're looking for. Remember, Wall Pilates builds overall strength, endurance, and fitness, but variety is the spice of life.

5. **Assess your nutrition and hydration:** Sometimes stalled progress happens because you're simply not giving your body what it needs to recover adequately from your workouts. Ensure you're eating enough protein to rebuild muscle along with fruits, vegetables, and healthy fats. Proper hydration is also key for energy levels, joint health, and muscle functioning, so drink enough water and electrolytes after workouts. Fuel your body properly to see results.

Stay consistent and be patient through plateaus. Small tweaks to challenge your body in new ways along with supporting your overall health will get you back on track toward your Wall Pilates goals.

Dealing with Persistent Pain and Discomfort

When exercising, it's normal to experience some muscle soreness or temporary discomfort. Building new muscles and repairing years of damage is hard work for your body so you can expect to experience a little bit of pain along the way. Having said that, persistent or sharp pain is a signal to stop and reassess your workouts and lingering pain typically means you've progressed too quickly or have poor form or alignment. Please, don't ignore it or "push through" when this happens as it can lead to injury. Instead, make use of the tips below and consult with a healthcare professional if none of the tips provided are effective after two full weeks.

1. **Identify the source of your pain:** Pinpoint exactly where the pain is coming from. Neck? Lower back? Shoulder? This helps determine the problematic exercise and appropriate modifications. Keep a journal noting activities that aggravate it, and ensure your form is correct, especially when doing movements that are on the floor.

2. **Change your alignment:** Everyone's bodies are different. We've experienced different injuries and compensated in different ways as we've moved through our lives. While alignment suggestions are important, the fact of the matter is that not everyone will be able to properly align their bodies, especially in the beginning phases of a new workout program. Make sure you're comfortably aligned, record yourself to check the form, and make small adjustments along the way. These small adjustments will add up, eventually leading to proper form.

3. **Take a step back:** Sometimes, pain and extended recovery time are an indication that you've advanced too quickly or that you're taking on more than your body can handle right now. Take a step back, opting to do fewer reps. Alternatively, lower any resistance or weight you've added to your workouts and make sure you are properly recovered between workouts.

4. **Isolate where it hurts the most:** Sometimes you can suffer from deferred pain, where a certain area feels tender but an injury originates from somewhere else. Make sure that you're properly assessing exactly what is causing your pain and pinpoint the muscle group. If pain is persistent in one area, seek a medical opinion and allow the joint or muscle to fully recover.

5. **Try massage, ice, and heat treatments:** To help speed up recovery, it's a good idea to try holistic-type treatments using hot or cold packs, or by booking yourself a massage. Massage and hot-cold treatments promote blood flow to areas of injury or recovery and help to relax overworked or injured muscles by reducing inflammation.

When dealing with injuries and pain, it's important to listen to your body, take some downtime to recover, and make sure you're not exacerbating the issue at hand. Some temporary soreness is a given but prolonged and/or sharp pain is an indication of a deeper issue you will need to address. When this happens, assess, scale back, and work on improving form. Injuries take time to heal so be patient.

Adjusting Workouts During Illness or Recovery

We live in a much smaller world where global travel and soaring populations mean we are more likely to pick up viruses and get sick. Added to this, we may need to recover from accidental injury. When this happens, we need to be mindful of our bodies and make the necessary modifications needed to accommodate what is happening and ensure we don't come to an abrupt workout halt.

Having said that, never engage in intensive exercise if you are experiencing upper respiratory illness, listen to your body, and stop any exercise immediately if you're feeling dizzy or you feel like your heart is being overworked. Stick to gentle warm-up stretches, engage in deep breathing, and rest your body as much as possible.

1. **Become in tune with your body**: Fatigue, pain, nausea, or breathing issues are all signals your body is sending you to stop or slow down while it fights off an infection and recovers. Never push through when you're feeling sick. Take time off, rest, hydrate, and nourish your body. Check in with your healthcare provider about when a good time to resume training would be.

2. **Start slow and build intensity**: While recovering, it's important to reduce the intensity of your workouts for about a week and then slowly build up the intensity and duration of each workout session. This allows you to transition your body from illness or injury to strength in a healthier way.

3. **Reduce your workouts**: For less serious illnesses and injuries, you may want to consider cutting back the number of exercise sessions you would normally have. Scale back to two or three workouts and make sure these are light, easy-to-do sessions.

4. **Slow down on complementary exercises**: It's important to keep up with your cardiovascular health but you don't want to place your heart under unnecessary strain. A slow, leisurely walk can't do you any harm if you're not overly fatigued but this is not the time to engage in vigorous activities or get into a swimming pool.

5. **Place more focus on circulatory stretches**: Full body, deep movements will help stimulate blood circulation and speed up recovery. Wide motions like cat/cow stretches, and hip circles aren't taxing on the body and work with the body's natural healing processes.

When you're ill or recovering, it's very important that you adjust your diet to help support recovery. This means incorporating nutrient-dense foods that are easy to digest, like soups and broths. Up your vitamin C intake by opting for freshly squeezed citrus fruits, and make sure that you're staying well hydrated.

The key to a quicker recovery is to be intuitive and listen to your body. Adapt your workouts accordingly and take time off if need be. There is absolutely no shame in a week or two of rest and recovery for the greater good of a healthy body. Once you're able to, you can get back to your workouts. The beauty of muscle memory is that time off doesn't mean taking a step back in progress and your body will remember what it's meant to do when the time is right.

Modifying Exercises for Different Fitness Levels

Wall Pilates is accessible to everyone, regardless of physical limitations. In fact, I've seen wheelchair-bound people engaging in a healthy, active life by using Wall Pilates as a way to strengthen their upper bodies. As mentioned before, Wall Pilates can be safely and effectively adapted with the right modifications allowing just about everyone the opportunity to get stronger and healthier.

Limitations aside, as you progress with your Wall Pilates workouts, you may find that each of the movements isn't as challenging. Modifications don't only apply to physical limitations but to the intensity of your workout too. Take a look at the advice below for more information on how you can modify your Wall Pilates workouts.

- Increase or decrease your resistance: Matching your strength and endurance with varying levels of resistance will ensure you're getting the best out of your workout. Add resistance bands or hand weights for a more challenging workout or move closer to the wall for a less intense workout.

- Deepen or lessen your range of motion: You can limit or extend your range of movement depending on your mobility and flexibility. Lower fitness and flexibility levels can try to perform partial movements, extending their range of motion as they improve over time. For more advanced workouts, try to increase your range of motion and begin moving fluidly from one movement to the next.

- Modify your repetitions and duration: Fewer and more reps, and including additional workouts will tailor-make your workout. Beginners can try to set the benchmark at 5 reps while more advanced people can increase their reps to

10. Once 10 reps become achievable, you can move on to sets, extending your workout from 1 set to 2 sets, and then 3 sets of each workout.

- Alter your transitions: In the beginning, you may need to take breaks between each movement but as you progress, you can begin to seamlessly transition between each of your exercises. This may shorten the duration of your workouts but will still provide an intense workout as a whole. Once you are able to complete a workout from start to finish without a break, you can consider adding more repetitions and sets to each workout.

- Support yourself: Using extra props like a chair, a sturdy piece of furniture, a pillow, a balance ball, or knee padding can really help with the precision of your movements. Added to that, props can ensure you don't get injured while building up your strength and flexibility.

The key to any modification is to work within your current limitations while still making sure to push your body in a healthy way. Progressing too quickly can mean you open yourself up to injury but slow progress can mean plateaus. As with any exercise program, balance is key, and learning to listen to your body, accepting there will be down days, and ensuring you're taking the time to celebrate each of your small wins is critical to gradual progress.

After all, perfecting your technique and showing up every day to complete a workout that fits within your current limitations is far more important than pushing yourself to progress quickly. Trust that consistency is what is needed to build strength, flexibility, and balance.

When in doubt, remember to place your workouts on pause and speak to a professional who can help you understand what is happening with your body. Trial and error is a great companion but if you're experiencing more issues than progress, it's important to find out why.

Conclusion

Moving Forward—Maintaining Your Wall Pilates Practices and Embracing Change

Entering into the years after 50 is one that can come with change and limitations but it is also a journey through conscious wellness practices. As we age, it's vital that we begin thinking about sustainability and consistency when it comes to our budding health and wellness practices. The initial enthusiasm and excitement around starting something new will eventually fade, and we'll be faced with the true test—can we maintain these small but potent daily rituals that nourish our bodies and spirits in the long run?

This final chapter is dedicated to you—our reader who has decided to embrace Wall Pilates and a healthy life. Of course, life brings with it inevitable ebbs and flows and it's important that you are prepared to let go of any rigid expectations around "perfect" practices and consistency. Instead, you need to understand that some weeks your schedule will allow daily Wall Pilates sessions, and other times, you'll be grateful for two brief workouts. The same applies to your diet—no one is saying you shouldn't enjoy your life or eat a cake or two. What is important as you age is to release yourself from self-judgment and learn to embrace your commitment to a consistent and joyful new era of your life.

If you're going to maintain your motivation long-term it's critical that you care for your body and honor just how incredible it is. You will need to develop an acceptance for the phase of your life you're in and understand that your age and your ability to take control of the aging process is the ultimate reward!

For many of us, this acceptance doesn't come easily. We forget to have fun with our routines and admonish ourselves for a lack of progress—stuck in comparisons of what was possible 20, 30, or even 40 years prior.

The cold hard reality is that we cannot move backward in life and all we have is this moment, right now, so put on your favorite song, switch up your workouts, and stay curious, engaged, and appreciative of where you are in your journey right now!

So what can you expect to learn from this final chapter?

We're going to take you through how to set long-term goals at an age when you don't have 60 years of active living left and show you how to embrace your body as it undergoes each of the natural aging processes. Added to this, we'll introduce you to different Pilates disciplines that are designed and developed for your 50-plus body. We'll show you how with the addition of some simple at-home equipment, you can spice up your Wall Pilates workouts, and the chapter will end with acceptance, confidence, and vitality—key components for the years to come.

Getting older certainly doesn't mean having to let go of our goals and dreams. It simply means setting new goals and reaching for new starts along the way. Together, we can explore how to move forward and embrace change for a long, beautiful, and strong life. While aging brings inevitable changes, practicing Wall Pilates equips us with the tools (and strength) we need to embrace this next life phase with energy, purpose, and self-assurance. By cultivating physical vitality along with mental fortitude, we greet aging with confidence to continue pursuing what sets our spirit alight.

Before continuing with your Wall Pilates journey, I'd like to ask you to leave me feedback and a review on your experience with this book and how it revolutionized your life. Creating books that help people like you is my passion and purpose and your feedback is absolutely invaluable to my craft.

Now, all that is left to do is trust that committing to Wall Pilates gives you the tools needed to greet this gift of aging with grace, command over your capabilities, and wisdom to cherish it all. Feel empowered to live with joy, move with freedom, and embrace this season with confidence from within.

Exercise Index